Theoretical Basis *of* Occupational Therapy
Second Edition

Mary Ann McColl, PhD
Queen's University
Kingston, Ontario

Mary Law, PhD
McMaster University
Hamilton, Ontario

Debra Stewart, MSc
McMaster University
Hamilton, Ontario

Lorna Doubt, MSc
Cobourg, Ontario

Nancy Pollock, MSc
McMaster University
Hamilton, Ontario

Terry Krupa, PhD
Queen's University
Kingston, Ontario

with assistance on historical chapters by
Penny Bryden, PhD
Mount Allison University
Sackville, New Brunswick

SLACK
INCORPORATED

An innovative information, education, and management company
6900 Grove Road • Thorofare, NJ 08086

The author, editor, and publisher cannot accept responsibility for errors or exclusions or for the out-come of the application of the material presented herein. There is no expressed or implied warranty of this book or information imparted by it.

The work SLACK publishes is peer reviewed. Prior to publication, recognized leaders in the field, educators, and clinicians provide important feedback on the concepts and content that we publish. We welcome feedback on this work.

Care has been taken to ensure that drug selection, dosages, and treatments are in accordance with currently accepted/recommended practice. Due to continuing research, changes in government poli-cy and regulations, and various effects of drug reactions and interactions, it is recommended that the reader review all materials and literature provided for each drug use, especially those that are new or not frequently used.

Library of Congress Cataloging-in-Publication Data

The theoretical basis of occupational therapy / Mary Ann McColl ... [et al.] ; with assistance on historical chapters from Penny Bryden.-- 2nd ed.
    p. ; cm.
Includes bibliographical references and indexes.
  ISBN 1-55642-540-6 (pbk. : alk. paper)
  1. Occupational therapy.
  [DNLM: 1. Occupational Therapy. WB 555 T396 2003] I. McColl, Mary Ann,
  RM735 .T47 2003
  615.8'515--dc21

                                                                        2002008062
Printed in the United States of America.
Published by: SLACK Incorporated
                         6900 Grove Road
                         Thorofare, NJ 08086-9447 USA
                         Telephone: 856-848-1000
                         Fax: 856-853-5991
                         www.slackbooks.com

Contact SLACK Incorporated for more information about other books in this field or about the availability of our books from distributors outside the United States.

Contents

About the Authors

Mary Ann McColl, PhD is a professor in occupational therapy at Queen's University in Kingston, Ontario, and director of research at Queen's Centre for Health Services and Policy Research. She was formerly the head of occupational therapy at Queen's, and before that she was director of research at Lyndhurst Spinal Cord Centre, Toronto, Ontario, and assistant professor in occupational therapy at the University of Toronto. She is one of the authors of the *Canadian Occupational Performance Measure*, as well as several other books, including *Introduction to Disability* (McColl & Bickenbach, 1998).

Mary Law, PhD is a professor and associate dean of rehabilitation science, associate member of the Department of Clinical Epidemiology and Biostatistics, and co-director of CanChild Centre for Childhood Disability Research at McMaster University, Hamilton, Ontario. Her clinical and research interests centre on the development and validation of client-centred outcome measures, evaluation of occupational therapy interventions with children, the effect of environmental factors on the participation of children with disabilities in day-to-day activities, and transfer of research knowledge into practice.

Debra Stewart, MSc is an assistant clinical professor in the School of Rehabilitation Science and a co-investigator of CanChild Centre for Childhood Disability Research. She also provides private, community-based occupational therapy services to children and youth with special needs as part of REACH Therapy Services.

Lorna Doubt, MSc has been an adjunct lecturer in School of Rehabilitation Therapy at Queen's University and is currently a paediatric therapy consultant for Northumberland Child Development Centre, Port Hope, and case manager for Northern Lights Vocational Services, Minden, Ontario.

Nancy Pollock, MSc is associate clinical professor, School of Rehabilitation Science and co-investigator, CanChild Centre for Childhood Disability Research. Her research, teaching, and clinical practice focus on children and adolescents with developmentally related occupational performance problems. She is also one of the authors of the *Canadian Occupational Performance Measure*.

Terry Krupa, PhD is an assistant professor and chair of the Occupational Therapy Program at Queen's University. Her research interests focus on the processes by which individuals with psychiatric disabilities come to participate in meaningful community occupations. Dr. Krupa is also involved in examining interpretations of disability and how this influences service delivery.

Penny Bryden, PhD is an associate professor and Head of the Department of History at Mount Allison University. She is the author of *Planners and Politicians: Liberal Politics and Social Policy, 1957-1968*, which is about the design and introduction of a national Medicare program in Canada.

Preface

We are very pleased to be able to offer this second edition of *Theoretical Basis of Occupational Therapy*, and grateful for the opportunity to implement some of the ideas we have learned from teaching theory to occupational therapy students in the last 10 years, since the first edition was released.

Like the previous edition, this book has a number of aims:

- To assemble occupational therapy theory for ease of access
- To organize occupational therapy theory in a way that makes sense to occupational therapists
- To propose a way of filing, storing, and using theory to support practice in occupational therapy
- To promote life-long learning in occupational therapy theory

The book uses two metaphors, the *filing cabinet* and the *toolbox*, to suggest ways that occupational therapists may organize, sort, store, and retrieve theoretical tools that assist them in practice.

Readers who are familiar with the first edition will notice a number of improvements in this edition:

- The opening chapters are expanded to better explain how theory may be used in occupational therapy.
- Three central ideas in occupational therapy are developed throughout the book—that occupation is essential to human health, that occupation changes, and that occupation can be used as a therapeutic tool.
- The annotated bibliography chapters (7 through 13) are organized by theory area, rather than chronologically. This facilitates access to related literature in a particular area.
- The concepts of change and therapeutic applications are addressed in this edition.
- Chapters 7 through 13 contain references to theory found in books as well as journals.

This edition focuses on the years from 1975 to 2000, a 25-year period over which occupational therapy theory developed and expanded quickly and prodigiously. It was also a period during which occupational therapy theory consolidated its focus on occupation as the defining construct. We encourage readers interested in theory prior to 1975 to continue to consult the first edition. It remains a useful resource for theory published in the first three-quarters of the 20th century.

We hope in presenting this second edition that we have been able to communicate not only our respect for the early theorists and their ideas, but also our excitement about recent developments in occupational therapy theory. We have emphasized the history of occupational therapy theory to illustrate the depth of the intellectual tradition associated with occupational therapy. We have attempted to trace ideas to their origins, whether in occupational therapy or in other disciplines, and to track the creative intellectual process involved in the development of theory up to the present day. On behalf of all the authors, I invite you to join us in exploring and discovering the depth and breadth of occupational therapy theory.

—*Mary Ann McColl, PhD*

1 INTRODUCTION
A BASIS FOR THEORY IN OCCUPATIONAL THERAPY

Mary Ann McColl, PhD

This is a textbook about occupational therapy theory. Occupational therapy theory provides us with ways of thinking about occupation and about the kinds of things that can affect occupation. Our purpose is not to advance a new theory or advocate for a particular existing theory, but rather to offer a way to gather, organize, and analyze the growing body of theory in occupational therapy.

The purpose of theory in occupational therapy is twofold:

1. To understand humans and their occupations

2. To be able to predict and change human functioning and occupational performance

The central construct that defines and unites occupational therapy theory is *occupation*. We use this term not in the colloquial sense, which refers to one's vocation, job, or field of professional expertise. Instead, we use occupation in the historical sense, referring to all aspects of daily living that contribute to health and fulfilment for an individual.

Occupation is used throughout this book to refer to purposeful or meaningful activities in which humans engage as part of their normal daily lives. Occupation is the touchstone that helps to focus the practice of occupational therapy, and it is the overarching idea that gives unity and meaning to the theory base of occupational therapy.

Throughout the literature in occupational therapy, three ideas or themes are repeated. These three ideas have become the basis for the development of the profession of occupational therapy. These include the ideas that:

1. Occupation is a basic feature of all human beings, essential to health.

2. Human occupation changes to meet internal and external demands on the individual.

3. Occupation can be structured, manipulated, and used to remediate occupational dysfunction.

The remainder of this chapter, as well as four additional chapters (5, 6, 7, and 14), will expand these three ideas.

Occupation is Essential for Human Health

Occupation is comprised of three areas: self-care, productivity, and leisure. Each is undertaken in a balance that is consistent with health and that is satisfying to the individual:

✖ *Self-care* includes activities that the individual performs for the purpose of maintaining the self in a condition that allows for function. In other words, it typically includes activities of daily and community living.

✖ *Productivity* refers to the activities that customarily fill the bulk of one's day and which contribute to economic preservation, home and family maintenance, and service or personal development. There is a component of obligation attached to productivity. In its most traditional form, productivity takes the form of salaried employment. However, it may also include work around one's home or voluntary work on the condition that some commitment or obligation is implied in the performance of these duties. It may also include child care or other care-giving. Productivity may include those initiatives taken on by an individual in preparation for future productivity. These include developmental play in young children and education or training at older ages. Productive activities often represent our contribution to our home, family, community, workplace, or society. They validate our need to be useful and to feel that we accomplish something within our own sphere of influence.

✖ *Leisure* includes activities that one engages in when one is freed from the obligation to be productive. Leisure activities are defined by the personal preferences and interests of the individual. They may be sedentary or active, social or individual, creative or technical. They are usually voluntary in nature and fully discretionary. They often allow us to express a creative or personal side of ourselves that does not find expression in our other daily activities.

We have observed that the theoretical literature in occupational therapy most commonly identifies occupation as a function of the person on one hand and the environment on the other (Canadian Asssociaton of Occupational Therapists [CAOT], 1997; Law et al., 1996; McColl, 1998; McColl, Law, & Stewart, 1992). The individual is further broken down into a number of components, which correspond to systems in the body. The most common components used to describe the individual include physical, psychological-emotional, cognitive-neurological, and socio-cultural (CAOT, 1981; McColl, Law, & Stewart, 1992; Reed, 1984). Figure 1-1 offers a generic model of occupation that serves as a basis for occupational therapy theory.

Each of these components (personal and environmental) contributes to the successful execution of occupation. Furthermore, a problem in any of these areas can interfere with successful, satisfying, meaningful human occupation.

The *physical* component of the person refers to musculoskeletal capacities. The physical determinants of occupation include strength, range of motion, and endurance. In order to understand occupation from the perspective of the physical component, we require a physical analysis of strengths and deficits, and the extent to which these can facilitate or interfere.

The *psychological-emotional* component of the person refers to both thoughts and feelings; that is, the intrinsic and learned responses of individuals to internal and external stimuli. From this perspective, successful occupational performance is predicated on healthy psychological and emotional responses toward the aspects of occupation that make up one's life.

The *cognitive-neurological* component refers to the central processing of internal and

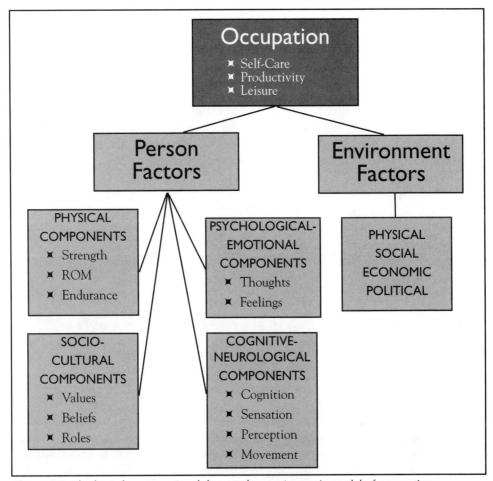

Figure 1-1. The basis for occupational therapy theory: A generic model of occupation.

external stimuli. Cognitive-neurological determinants of occupation include the cognitive, sensory, perceptual, and neurological integration of input essential to one's ability to carry out daily activities with success and satisfaction. The cognitive-neurological component is distinguishable from the physical component in that it focuses on the central nervous system, whereas the physical component focuses on peripheral, musculoskeletal functioning. It also differs from the psychological-emotional component in that it emphasizes the ability to process incoming information, rather than the psychological or emotional experience of it.

The *socio-cultural* component includes learned beliefs, attitudes, roles, and behaviours that are a result of socialization or upbringing. Socio-cultural determinants of occupation refer to the process of organizing one's occupation into social patterns or habits that conform to the social and cultural roles one fulfils. Occupational dysfunction occurs when performance and expectations diverge. Concepts are classified as socio-cultural determinants that are socially defined, constructed, or mediated. Therefore, concepts like time, roles, meaning, and spirituality may be considered parts of the socio-cultural component.

Finally, the *environment* is defined broadly to include both the physical and the social environments. We also typically think of three levels of environment: the micro-environment, referring to one's home and those with whom one lives; the meso-environment, referring to one's community, workplace, or neighbourhood; and the macro-environment, referring to the society in which one participates. The environmental determinants of occupation include any aspect of the environment that has the potential to either facilitate or impede occupation. Occupational dysfunction arising from the environmental component would be the result of an inadequate, an overly controlling, a hostile, or perhaps simply an indifferent environment.

Figure 1-1 defines and elaborates occupation for the purposes of this book. The ideas expressed in the model are not new ideas, but they are combined in a new way. They include ideas originally described by Meyer, Reilly, Reed, Yerxa, and both the American and Canadian Associations of Occupational Therapists. The model provides a generic framework for the theory of occupation, and a starting point from which to explore the various theories, perspectives and ideas that underlie occupational therapy. The model does not, in itself, represent a new theory of occupation or occupational therapy. Rather, it represents a definition of occupation, culled from a variety of sources. Chapters 7 and 8 deal further with the literature on occupation and health.

Occupation Changes to Meet Internal and External Demands

The literature in occupational therapy repeatedly refers to three processes through which human occupation changes: development, adaptation, and accommodation.

- *Developmental changes* in occupation occur when an external or internal demand sets in motion an intrinsically programmed change that is sequential and predictable.

- *Adaptative changes* in occupation occur when an external or internal demand elicits a behaviour that was perhaps previously successful but is now inadequate. In an effort to achieve mastery within the environment, new exploratory behaviours are attempted and are either reinforced or discouraged in terms of their success in achieving the desired effect.

- *Occupation* also changes in response to accommodations or changes in the environment aimed at enhancing the potential to support occupation.

Chapter 8 deals in detail with these three processes and the developments in our knowledge and understanding of them.

Occupation Can Be Used Therapeutically

Finally, there are three ways in which occupation can be structured and used therapeutically to effect optimum occupational performance. Remediation, compensation, and advocacy are processes through which occupational therapists interact with people seeking to make changes in occupation:

- *Remediation* refers to efforts aimed at fixing the problem by improving some aspect of the individual. For example, remediation would include using vigorous and prolonged activities to increase stamina and endurance.

- *Compensation* refers to efforts aimed at working around a problem by using other components of the individual or the environment to improve occupation. Some examples

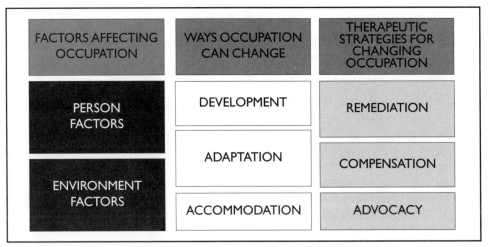

Figure 1-2. How occupation changes and how it may be used therapeutically.

of compensation include the application of technology, the marshalling of supports, and the modification of methods.

✷ *Advocacy* refers to initiatives taken by a therapist on behalf of a client, to pursue a change in the environment that will ultimately enhance occupation. For example, advocacy might include renegotiating roles with family members, providing education and training to employers, or consulting with policy makers.

Figure 1-2 attempts to show the relationships among the three basic ideas about occupation. Here are some basic tenets about occupation and occupational therapy that can be drawn from Figure 1-2:

✷ There are two types of factors affecting occupation: *person factors* and *environment factors*.

✷ Person factors can be changed through development and through adaptation.

✷ Environment factors can be changed through adaptation (proximal to the person) and accommodation (distal to the person).

✷ Therapeutic strategies used to bring about change vary depending on the type of change being sought.

✷ Remedial strategies may be used to bring about changes in development or adaptation; that is, the problem itself can be "fixed" through development (simulating the natural developmental process) or adaptation (learning through feedback from the environment).

✷ Compensatory strategies may be used to promote adaptation, while advocacy is the strategy typically used to achieve accommodation.

✷ Remedial and compensatory strategies may be used to address person factors.

✷ Compensation and advocacy may be used to bring about changes in environmental factors.

References

Canadian Association of Occupational Therapists. (1981). *Guidelines for the client-centred practice of occupational therapy*. Ottawa, ON: Supply & Services Canada.

Canadian Association of Occupational Therapists. (1997). *Enabling occupation*. Ottawa, ON: CAOT ACE.

Law, M., Cooper, B., Strong, S. Stewart, D., Rigby, P., & Letts, L. (1996). The Person-Environment-Occupation Model: A transactive approach to occupational performance. *Canadian Journal of Occupational Therapy, 63,* 9-23.

McColl, M. A. (1998). What do we need to know to practice occupational therapy in the community? *Am J Occup Ther, 52,* 11-8.

McColl, M. A., Law, M., & Stewart, D. (1992). *Theoretical basis of occupational therapy*. Thorofare, NJ: SLACK Incorporated.

Reed, K. (1984). *Models of practice in occupational therapy*. Baltimore: Williams & Wilkins.

<table>
<tr><td>2</td></tr>
</table>

THE OCCUPATIONAL THERAPY TOOLBOX
USES OF THEORY IN OCCUPATIONAL THERAPY

Mary Ann McColl, PhD

Theory is probably most easily understood as a tool for thinking. Thus, one's store of theory knowledge can be thought of as a toolbox, from which one selects the most appropriate tool for the job. Just like in carpentry:

✖ Tools do not do the job by themselves, but they assist us to do it.

✖ It is possible to use a number of different tools to do the same job; however, the correct tool does the job best and makes it easiest.

✖ Conversely, one tool may have applications in a variety of different situations.

✖ Different workers will have preferences for particular tools with which they are most comfortable and familiar.

✖ Some people try to use the same tool for every application. For example, many people use a screwdriver to take the lid off a paint tin, to pry two surfaces apart, or to scrape off old paint.

✖ On the other hand, people commonly use a knife or dime to do the job of a screwdriver.

✖ If the only tool you have is a hammer, it is amazing how every problem begins to look like a nail!

The carpentry metaphor demonstrates the flexibility of tools, but it also shows how tools become compromised when used in applications for which they were not intended.

In the same way, we can refer to the broad array of occupational therapy theory as *the tools of our practice*. Therefore, a toolbox is needed to organize and classify items, making it easier for therapists to find the right tool for every job. The toolbox is a repository from which occupational therapists can select ideas, concepts, and principles that help them to understand and influence the occupational performance of their clients. In this book, these ideas, concepts, and principles are referred to collectively as *theory*. We distinguish between:

✖ *Small-t theory*—a term that we use to refer collectively to ideas that help occupational therapists to think about and conceptualize what they do.

✖ *Large-T theory*—meaning a formalized, systematic representation of phenomena, complete with research evidence. Its purpose is to allow us to predict or anticipate relationships among concepts.

In this book, we use the more inclusive *small-t theory* to capture as many as possible of the important ideas or tools for thinking that occupational therapists can depend on in their daily practice.

Some theory is more appropriate for specific occupational problems than for others, and most occupational therapists have their favorite theoretical approaches. The choice of a favorite theoretical approach may be influenced by a number of factors, such as the area in which one practices, the theoretical approaches used by colleagues, the theories that were prevalent when one was educated, or the accessibility of particular theoretical literature, workshops, or continuing education opportunities.

Our occupational therapy toolbox is separated into two main sections: tools to help us understand occupation and tools to help us change occupation. The former offers us *ways to think* and the latter offers us *ways to act*. We typically call these two main categories of theory *conceptual models* and *models of practice*. Conceptual models help us to think about occupation and are typically made up of principles or statements about the relationship between occupation and other concepts. Models of practice help us act therapeutically to change occupation and are typically made up of assessment and intervention approaches. Ideally, there should be relationships between conceptual models and models of practice. That is, we should be able to trace the link between a practice approach and the conceptual ideas upon which it is based. Assessments and intervention approaches should clearly reflect the understanding of occupation and human health upon which they are based. Sensory integration is a good example of this. The conceptual model associated with sensory integration gives us theory to explain the relationship between incoming sensory input and occupational output. The model of practice associated with sensory integration offers us assessment tools and intervention modalities and techniques that apply the conceptual model or that instruct us how to act therapeutically according to the sensory integration approach. These practice tools are meant to allow us to assess and treat different types of sensory input to produce predictable changes in occupation.

The occupational therapy toolbox, or knowledge base, is further divided into two more sections: theory that is explicitly about occupation and theory that is generally about human beings and their environments. We will refer to these as occupational theory and basic theory. *Occupational theory* is specifically about occupation, and it is most often developed by occupational therapists. It attempts to explain occupation in relation to a variety of other factors, which are described further in the next chapter. *Basic theory* is all of the other theory, usually from other disciplines, that we learn and use to help us understand human beings in context. For example, our anatomy, physiology, biology, pathology, kinesiology, and other basic biomedical sciences help us to understand the physical aspect of the human being.

The distinction between occupational and basic theory is important. Those theoretical ideas classified as occupational theory describe occupation, each from its own particular perspective. For example, Mosey's *Recapitulation of Ontogenesis* would be considered occupational theory, since it explains the development of occupation and discusses specific occupational tasks (such as vocational choice and self-care) from a developmental perspective. On the other hand, developmental theories like those developed by Piaget and Erikson would be considered basic theories, since they discuss the development of human being and of specific human components, like cognition and social relationships. Basic theories, then,

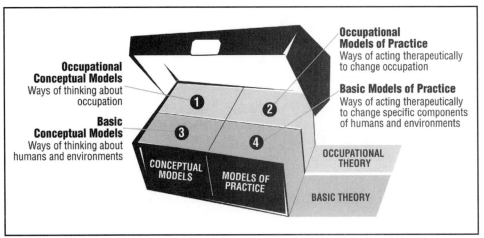

Figure 2-1. The occupational therapy toolbox.

are those theories that describe the components necessary for the development of occupation, such as cognitive development, physical development, social development, and so on, but which do not address occupation directly.

The occupational therapy toolbox, therefore, has four sections, like the matrix in Figure 2-1:

1. Theory located in section 1 of the toolbox includes conceptual models that help us to understand occupation and the things that interfere with occupation to produce problems. For example, theories about how occupation is acquired and how developmental factors can affect the acquisition of occupation would be found in the occupational conceptual models section.

2. Theory found in section 2 includes conceptual models from other disciplines that help us understand human beings in general. These do not deal specifically with occupation but rather with the components of people and environments (which admittedly influence occupation). For example, basic conceptual models about how muscles receive messages from the central nervous system to produce human movement would be found in section 2 of the occupational therapy toolbox.

3. Theory found in section 3 includes occupational therapy models of practice. This is theory that helps us to know how to act to help clients to improve their occupation. As an example, theory about how the environment may be modified to enhance occupation would be found in section 3, occupational models of practice.

4. Finally, theory found in section 4 of the matrix includes models of practice relating to specific components of humans and their environments. For example, theory about how occupational therapists might intervene with physical modalities to promote activity tolerance and endurance would be considered a basic model of practice.

In this textbook, we will focus on theory from the first quadrant of the toolbox: the occupational conceptual models. These are theories that, over the past century, have helped us to understand what occupation is and what factors affect it. Wherever possible, we will offer examples of theories that would be classified in one of the other quadrants of the toolbox: occupational models of practice or basic theory. However, the purpose of this book is to search out, identify, and classify theory that explains the phenomenon of occupation.

We have chosen the language for this book in a very purposeful fashion in an attempt to:

- Avoid a proliferation of terminology

- Use language that is descriptive and meaningful

- Use terms that are already in our lexicon and avoid the coining of new terms

- Be consistent and predictable in the use of language

To that end, we offer four terms and their definitions that will be used throughout this book:

- Conceptual models—ways of thinking about and understanding phenomena

- Models of practice—ways of acting therapeutically to make a change

- Occupational theory—theory dealing with occupation

- Basic theory—theory dealing with humans and their environments

THE OCCUPATIONAL THERAPY FILING CABINET

ORGANIZING OCCUPATIONAL THERAPY THEORY

3

Mary Ann McColl, PhD

Throughout our careers, first as students then as occupational therapists, we continually acquire knowledge concerning humans and their occupations in the areas described in Chapter 2. We perpetually add to and refine our understanding of occupation through:

* Experiences as occupational therapists
* Interactions with clients and their families
* Relationships with other professionals
* Continuing education, workshops, journals, and books

However, we do not always have a way of storing this knowledge so that it is readily accessible and usable. Imagine a huge cardboard box into which all of this knowledge is placed, piling up over a career of practicing and studying occupational therapy. Imagine having to rifle through that box each time we seek to understand a problem presented by a client, to provide a rationale for a particular therapeutic approach, or to explain occupational therapy to a client's family or to another professional.

Now imagine a filing cabinet in which you could file all of this information so that it was readily accessible and retrievable. How would you label the drawers of the filing cabinet? How would you organize the files contained in each drawer?

Figure 3-1 suggests a filing cabinet with five drawers, each one corresponding to one of the five determinants of occupation described in Chapter 1 (physical, psychological-emotional, cognitive-neurological, socio-cultural, and environmental, see Figure 1-1). In each drawer of the filing cabinet are four folders, corresponding to the four quadrants of the toolbox discussed in Chapter 2 (see Figure 2-1): occupational conceptual models, occupational models of practice, basic conceptual models, and basic models of practice. We contend that all of the knowledge, ideas, and theories used by occupational therapists can be readily classified in this filing cabinet.

The filing cabinet metaphor provides a classification system to organize the professional body of knowledge that we acquire as students and that we supplement and refine throughout our careers. Table 3-1 is a schematic diagram of the classification system. This system allows us to classify all of our basic occupational therapy education and to perpetually add,

Figure 3-1. A filing cabinet for occupational therapy theory.

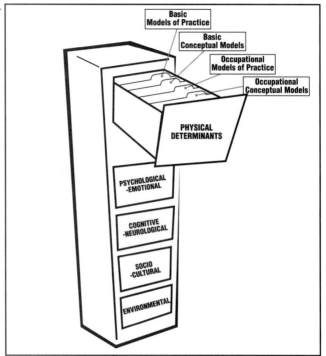

subtract, and alter content as our understanding of occupation changes and matures. The classification system is made up of five categories, corresponding to the five components of occupation outlined in Chapter 1: physical, psychological-emotional, cognitive-neurological, socio-cultural, and environmental. Within each category, we find occupational and basic theory, or theory pertaining directly to occupation and theory pertaining generally to humans and their environments. Furthermore, within each category we also find both conceptual models and models of practice.

Now let us look more closely at each of the five drawers of the filing cabinet and their contents. Each of these drawers, or theory areas, represents a way of understanding and analysing occupation and a way of identifying potentially remediable deficits that contribute to occupational dysfunction. For each drawer, the source of the problem in occupational functioning is different.

Physical Determinants of Occupation

- ✖ Theory pertaining to the physical determinants of occupation locates the problem interfering with occupation in the person and more specifically in the musculoskeletal system.

- ✖ Occupational conceptual models that would be classified here explain occupational problems in terms of deficits in physical functioning, particularly strength, range of motion, and endurance.

- ✖ Occupational models of practice filed in this drawer would strive to remediate occupation through the use of physical activities.

Table 3-1

A Taxonomy for Occupational Theory

	PERSON FACTORS				ENVIRONMENT FACTORS
	Physical	*Psychological-Emotional*	*Cognitive-Neurological*	*Socio-Cultural*	*Environmental*
Conceptual Models — *Occupational Conceptual Models*	Ways of thinking about the physical determinants of occupation (e.g., activity analysis, rehabilitative theory)	Ways of thinking about the psychological and emotional determinants of occupation (e.g., object-relations, personal causation)	Ways of thinking about the cognitive and neurological determinants of occupation (e.g., sensory integration, cognitive disabilities)	Ways of thinking about the social and cultural determinants of occupation (e.g., theory on habits, values, time)	Ways of thinking about the environmental determinants of occupation (e.g., person-environment-occupation, ecology of human perfection)
Basic Conceptual Models	Ways of thinking about the physical nature of human beings (e.g., anatomy, physiology)	E.g, psychology, psychiatry, neuro-psychiatry	E.g, motor control, sensory processing	E.g, anthropology, sociology	E.g., ecological theory, geography, urban planning, environmental press
Models of Practice — *Occupational Models of Practice*	Therapeutic strategies for dealing with physical impediments to occupation (e.g., graded activity, biomechanics, manual muscle testing, goniometry)	E.g, projective techniques, skills training	E.g., sensory integration, therapy, cognitive orientation to occupational performance	E.g, social skills, role analysis, habit training	Eg, ergonomics, universal design, assistive technology
Basic Models of Practice	Therapeutic strategies for altering the physical capacities of individuals (e.g., exercise)	E.g, Behavioural approach, psycho-educational therapy	E.g, NDT, PNF, Brunnstrom	E.g, family dynamics, role theory	E.g, urban planning

* Basic conceptual models filed in this drawer would include the basic physical sciences, such as anatomy, musculoskeletal physiology, kinesiology, and biomechanics.
* Basic models of practice involve the use of physical modalities to remediate strength, endurance, and range of motion.

Psychological-Emotional Determinants of Occupation

* Theory pertaining to the psychological and emotional determinants of occupation locates the problem interfering with occupation in the person's thoughts and feelings.
* Occupational conceptual models considered within this category explain occupational dysfunction in terms of the individual's feelings, attitudes, motivations, and coping resources for occupation.
* Occupational models of practice would include assessment and intervention methods to address the inherent meaning of occupation for the individual and a variety of approaches aimed at overcoming psychological obstacles to occupational function.
* Basic conceptual models arise from the disciplines of psychology, psychiatry, and neuropsychology.
* Basic models of practice instruct us about how to assess and treat underlying psychological problems, such as depression or anxiety.

Cognitive-Neurological Determinants of Occupation

* Theory pertaining to the cognitive-neurological determinants of occupation locates the problem interfering with occupation in the person, particularly in the central nervous system.
* Occupational conceptual models classified in this area explain the inability to perform daily occupation as a function of the individual's inability to experience, process, and apply incoming information. It is important here to recognize the distinctions between cognitive-neurological theory and both the physical and psychological emotional theories. Physical theory would be used to understand problems associated with peripheral damage to the nervous system, while cognitive-neurological theory would be used to understand problems associated with the central nervous system. Psychological-emotional theory would be used to understand thoughts and cognitive processes that are maladaptive, whereas cognitive-neurological theory would be used to understand the inability to engage in particular cognitive processes.
* Occupational models of practice are based on the assumption that successful occupational functioning may be achieved only when neurological and integrative capabilities are restored, and both intrinsic and extrinsic input can be meaningfully interpreted to allow appropriate occupational responses.
* Basic conceptual models in this area come from a number of other disciplines, including neuroanatomy, neurophysiology, and some aspects of neurobehavioural psychology.

✖ Basic models of practice include models developed by occupational therapists and others that do not refer specifically to occupation. Instead, they address the neurological system and its recovery from injury or illness. They focus specifically on the neurological mechanisms and processes. The assumption, of course, is that if the neurological structures necessary for occupation are in place, then occupational function will surely follow.

Socio-Cultural Determinants of Occupation

✖ Theory pertaining to the socio-cultural determinants of occupation locates the problem interfering with occupation in the person, more specifically in internalised social and cultural concepts.

✖ Occupational conceptual models falling into this category analyse occupation in terms of socially constructed phenomena, such as roles, habits, time use, and beliefs.

✖ Occupational models of practice generally aim at rationalizing expectations, demands and capabilities, and at structuring social roles and occupational activities to enhance success.

✖ Basic conceptual models come primarily from sociology and anthropology, and help us to understand how humans function within groups, communities, and societies.

✖ Basic models of practice come from social psychology and pertain to the treatment of individuals in contexts, groups, communities, and relationships.

Environmental Determinants of Occupation

✖ Theory pertaining to the environmental determinants of occupation locates the problem interfering with occupation, *not* in the person, but in the environment.

✖ Occupational conceptual models in this category attempt to understand occupation in terms of the environmental forces that act on it.

✖ Occupational models of practice within this framework are predicated on changes in the environment to facilitate occupation. Therefore, therapeutic efforts are directed at the environment, rather than at the client, and changes made as a result of therapy should be seen in the environment. This theoretical approach suggests a structural analysis of problems rather than an intrapersonal or interpersonal approach. Rehabilitation in general, and occupational therapy in particular, has historically focused primarily on the remediation of individuals. The environmental approach deals with the interaction of the individual and his or her surroundings.

✖ Basic conceptual models help us to understand the nature of environments and come from a variety of disciplines, including anthropology, sociology, geography, art, economics, and politics, as well as physics and biomechanics.

✖ Basic models of practice aim to change the environment, either through urban and social planning, advocacy, organizational tactics or other methods of structural change.

What gets classified in each of these drawers and folders? Ideas about:

1. What occupation is all about

2. What things can interfere with occupation

3. What happens to people when components fail

4. How occupational therapists can act to restore health and occupation

It should be emphasized here that these five theory areas need not be considered mutually exclusive of one another. A particular theoretical idea may be classified in more than one place, depending on its context or the details associated with its application. We should also note that some well-known theories may not fit tidily into one theory area—elements of it may fit best in different theory areas. For example, the Model of Human Occupation contains ideas from a number of different theory areas. Concepts like values, habits, and temporal adaptation fit well with the socio-cultural theory area, while ideas like personal causation, interests, and skill learning fit more comfortably in the psychological-emotional area. This should not detract from the credibility or effectiveness of either the taxonomy or the model. It is simply a product of the cross-section of two ways of looking at occupation. It is enormously beneficial in working with theory to be able to consider it from different perspectives and to be flexible in thinking about occupation.

We referred in the last chapter to *large-T theory* or named theory, and to *small-t theory*, or generic unnamed theory in occupational therapy. Particularly in the last 10 years, a number of named theories have emerged, such as the Model of Human Occupation, the Cognitive Disabilities Model, and the Person-Environment-Occupation Model. Usually a theory that merits a name is one that offers a systematic view of a particular domain; it purports to be a comprehensive, internally consistent theoretical tool. Very often, named theories also have a body of empirical evidence associated with them. They are structured such that it is possible to generate hypotheses from their stated principles and to test those hypotheses to support and validate the theory. They are intended to render the world more predictable and to permit generalization about relationships between concepts of interest. Usually, these theories are easily recognised as theory, because they are labeled.

However, equally important are ideas that guide and govern practice that are not incorporated into formal theoretical systems. For example, occupational therapists depend heavily on ideas about grading activity to present an increasing challenge toward mastery. This idea has been a part of occupational therapy's thinking and culture since the early part of this century and yet has never been associated with a particular author or named theory. As such, we refer to it as *small-t theory*, and consider it essential to capture in a book of this type. Another example of unnamed theory is the "4 P's" of energy conservation: posture, planning, pacing, and prioritising. This is an enormously useful intellectual tool or piece of theory about energy conservation, whose origins have been lost—it has become a part of the folk wisdom of occupational therapy. It does not have an author's name associated with it nor a body of research to support it, but this does not diminish its importance or utility in the consciousness and processes of occupational therapy. Therefore, we include it as theory, or as a tool for thinking, for the purpose of this book.

The taxonomy offers the opportunity to classify both types of theory and also offers the flexibility to use more than one theory area to cover all the important aspects of a particular theory. Table 3-1 illustrates how some named and unnamed theories are classified according to the taxonomy.

Using the Toolbox and the Filing Cabinet To Understand Occupation

4

Mary Ann McColl, PhD

We have talked up to this point about classifying theory so that it is more readily available to us. Now let us talk about how we can actually use theory. Perhaps the best way to illustrate the utility of the toolbox and the filing cabinet is with an example. The following example shows how we can use theory from all five areas of occupational therapy theory to help us:

1. Understand the occupational problem faced by the client

2. Understand the corresponding problems in underlying components of the person and the environment

3. Intervene to improve the functioning of a particular component

4. Intervene to improve occupation directly

> Lynn is a 27-year-old woman who has recently been hospitalized with suspected diagnosis of multiple sclerosis (MS) following an episode of weakness, fatigue, and visual changes. She is married with two small children, 3 years and 9 months. Her husband, Cliff, works long hours as a stockbroker. Her mother has come to stay and look after the children while Lynn is in the hospital. Lynn is a legal secretary. Her discharge is planned for the end of the week, and everyone is wondering how Lynn will manage at home and at work. In particular, there is a concern about how she will balance the occupational requirements of returning to work and caring for her children. An occupational therapy assessment is requested.

Using the Filing Cabinet

1. From the perspective of a therapist who functioned primarily from the *physical* theory area, Lynn's potential to fulfil her responsibilities at home and at work would be seen primarily as a function of her stamina and ability to cope with the physical demands of both jobs. The occupational therapy assessment would focus on Lynn's ability to fulfill the physical requirements of her occupational roles, particularly with regard to

endurance. Occupational therapy intervention might focus on remedial activities to increase Lynn's activity tolerance and compensatory strategies to save energy and optimize physical capacity.

2. A therapist functioning primarily from the *psychological-emotional* theory area would seek to understand Lynn's thoughts and feelings associated with returning home and resuming the dual functions of child care and work. Assessment would focus on how these feelings were affecting Lynn's occupation and possibly on the origins of these feelings and ideas. Occupational therapy intervention would offer strategies to cope with the feelings, perhaps attempting to raise them to a higher level of consciousness. Treatment may also provide problem-solving methods to prevent her feelings from interfering.

3. For someone whose primary method of understanding occupation was *cognitive-neurological* theory, Lynn's problems would be understood as potentially related to problems in processing incoming information, either cognitively, perceptually, or neurologically. This therapist would want to assess Lynn's capacity to process incoming information, to assess the extent of the neurological problem underlying Lynn's occupational dysfunction. Intervention would be consistent with neurological theories about multiple sclerosis.

4. The *socio-cultural* theory area offers another way to understand and address Lynn's occupational issues. Lynn's problems may be understood in terms of her roles as mother, wife, worker, daughter, and so on. Assessment would focus on Lynn's beliefs about the roles she plays, her expectations of herself in those roles, and her perceptions about the expectations of other key players. Occupational therapy intervention would seek to reconcile her role expectations and understand role behaviours, to structure her use of time, and to marshal resources and supports to fulfill these roles.

5. Finally, from the *environmental* perspective, Lynn's problems would be understood in terms of the ability of her environment to support her in her occupation. Assessment would focus on the physical environment (i.e., home and work) and the social environment (i.e., Lynn's husband, mother, friends, neighbours, and community services). Assessment would attempt to determine what supports and barriers the environment presented, and intervention would attempt to enhance supports and remove barriers.

The example illustrates a number of points:

✖ First, it shows that there are many different ways to approach any occupational problem. You may have thought of others that we have not presented.

✖ Second, it shows that ways of approaching occupational problems can be classified into the five theory areas that we have suggested.

✖ Third, the example shows that some ways of understanding a particular problem are more appropriate than others. For example, in our opinion, the physical, socio-cultural, and environmental approaches offer the most promise of achieving a meaningful understanding of Lynn's situation and of intervening in an effective manner. However, for therapists with a distinct preference and expertise in a particular theory area, the example shows how it is possible for that theory area to be applicable across a broad spectrum of clients and occupational problems.

✖ Fourth, the example shows how assessment and treatment dovetail within a particular theory area.

⚍ Finally, the example raises the issue of the boundaries that exist in each of the theory areas. In practice, it is uncommon for a therapist to practice using ideas from only one theory area. More often, we combine ideas and principles from a variety of theory areas. We often refer to this as an eclectic approach to practice. There is nothing wrong with an eclectic approach to practice, as long as it is not a euphemism for an atheoretical (i.e., a common sense or gut reaction) approach to practice. To ensure that this is not the case, it is important to be able to identify the origins of particular ideas that contribute to one's eclectic approach, and to ensure that the principles used or the assumptions underlying them are not fundamentally conflicting.

This process of generating hypotheses about factors affecting occupational problems leads us directly to the first quadrant of the toolbox: occupational conceptual models. Occupational conceptual models provide us with an understanding of the factors affecting occupation. In other words, this quadrant contains theory about the relationships between occupational problems and components of humans and environments.

Alternatively, we may say that the process of generating hypotheses for the origins of occupational problems leads us to the first folder in each drawer of the filing cabinet. In much the same way as we did in our example with Lynn, occupational therapists rifle through the first folder in each drawer of their mental filing cabinet to generate hypotheses about why people are experiencing the problems they see. Is there a physical impediment to occupation? Do thoughts or feelings (psychological-emotional), beliefs or values (socio-cultural) interfere with occupation? Is there a central processing problem that prevents the smooth transition between receiving sensory input and producing occupational output (cognitive-neurological)? Do the physical and social environments adequately support the occupation of the individual? Theory about each of these five areas will help us to develop several working hypotheses about the factors contributing to difficulties with occupation.

To follow on with Lynn's example, our hypotheses are that:

1. Multiple sclerosis has affected Lynn's physical capacity, particularly her strength and endurance. Lynn's physical capacity may not be adequate to meet the demands of her various occupations, and the physical demands of her occupations need to be considered in relation to their effects on her MS (physical theory). Therefore, the first step would be a comprehensive evaluation of the physical demands of her various occupations using theory about activity analysis.

2. Lynn may be expected to have a psychological reaction to her changed circumstances that could further affect her occupational performance (psychological-emotional theory). Classical occupational therapy theory about the importance of occupation and the potential of occupation to organize and consolidate identity would be important here.

3. Since MS is a condition of the central nervous system, we automatically think of the cognitive-neurological theory area to interpret Lynn's situation. We draw on our basic theory to understand the disease's effects on the nervous system and its impact on occupation. Further, we may use cognitive-neurological theory to understand the perceptual changes that Lynn reported and to explore ways of intervening.

4. Lynn may have difficulty reconciling and balancing roles in light of her activity limitations (socio-cultural theory). Lynn's occupation is impaired because of conflict among her various valued roles, and her inability to re-adjust the demands of these roles to her new status. Theory about the relationships of roles, values and habits to occupation might also be useful here.

5. There may be environmental impediments to optimal occupational functioning (environmental theory). Lynn may be experiencing expectations and demands from the environment that she does not feel she can meet, and she may or may not be receiving the required support to do so. Theory about the environment and its impact on occupation might help us to understand the role of the environment in Lynn's difficulties.

Using the Toolbox

To develop a fuller and more detailed understanding of each of these hypotheses, occupational therapists rely on theory about humans and their environments, usually originating in other disciplines. For example, to elaborate on the second hypothesis pertaining to Lynn, we might consult our psychology and psychiatry background to fill in what we know about psychological reactions to illness and disability. To follow the filing cabinet analogy, that would be found in the folder in the second drawer, which pertains to conceptual models about the psychological-emotional nature of human beings. For the third hypothesis, we might consult our basic conceptual models from sociology for information about roles and role conflict.

To better understand the nature of occupational problems, occupational therapists next proceed to find out more about the functioning of specific performance components underlying the most promising hypotheses. To understand the nature and extent of underlying problems, they rely on basic models of practice to suggest appropriate assessments of human performance components and of the environment.

In our example, we might use elements from various occupational models of practice such as activity analysis (physical determinants of occupation), an unstructured interview about expectations associated with discharge and return home, a role inventory, a measure of role conflict (socio-cultural theory), a home assessment, a support inventory, or interviews with other key personnel, such as husband and employer (environmental theory). We might also use elements from basic models of practice, such as a depression inventory, a self-esteem measure (psychological-emotional theory area), or perceptual or neurological testing (cognitive-neurological theory). Armed with all of this information and a thorough understanding of the nature, extent, and probable origins of the occupational problems, the therapist is finally ready to share the results of her assessment with the client and to work together to set goals while selecting therapeutic approaches to remediate occupational problems. For this task, she relies on models of practice to offer guidance for therapeutic approaches to occupational problems in each of the five areas of theory and on knowledge about how occupation changes and how therapists may contribute to the process of change.

Using the Taxonomy to Classify Occupational Conceptual Models

5

Mary Ann McColl, PhD

Chapters 7 through 13 of this book take the form of an annotated bibliography, whose purpose is to organize and compile the wealth of occupational therapy theory that has been produced in each of the five theory areas in the period between 1975 and 2000. This period has been a particularly rich and productive one for occupational therapy theory. It represents a new era in occupational therapy theory: one focussed on occupation as the central construct in occupational therapy. This book extends the theory coverage offered in the first edition, which ended with the year 1990.

The book focuses on occupational conceptual models. Thus, the emphasis of all of the articles listed in the Chapters 7 through 13 is to provide a new understanding of occupation or to contribute to our knowledge about occupation. In each chapter, examples of articles will be offered that might be classified in the second, third, and fourth quadrants of the toolbox (occupational models of practice, basic conceptual models, or basic models of practice). However, the extensive bibliographic entries will be restricted to occupational conceptual models (quadrant 1 of the toolbox).

The theory in which we are interested is found throughout professional periodicals and textbooks produced in the years between 1975 and 2000. A complete list of the journals consulted to develop the bibliography is contained in Table 5-1. The list includes 12 journals from five countries. In addition, a number of textbooks have been included in recognition of the fact that much of our theory over the period is best covered in textbooks developed for occupational therapy students. Where multiple editions of a book are available, both the first and the most recent will be emphasized. A complete list of criteria used to select theory is presented in Table 5-2. While significant efforts were made to identify and review all important theory in each of the pertinent chapters, there may be readers who feel that particular entries have been incorrectly classified or entirely overlooked. For any oversights, we apologise. We have attempted to apply the criteria fairly and equitably, however we recognize that the bibliography is not exhaustive.

In this book, we hope to avoid entanglement in terminology about theory and the evolution of another set of definitions and theoretical terminology. As discussed in Chapter 2, we propose to use the word *theory* in its broadest and most generic sense: to mean concep-

Table 5-1 Journals Included in the Annotated Bibliography

American Journal of Occupational Therapy
Australian Occupational Therapy Journal
British Journal of Occupational Therapy
Canadian Journal of Occupational Therapy
Journal of Occupational Science
Occupational Therapy International
Occupational Therapy Journal of Research
Occupational Therapy in Mental Health
Occupational Therapy in Health Care
Physical and Occupational Therapy in Paediatrics
Physical and Occupational Therapy in Geriatrics
Scandanavian Journal of Occupational Therapy

Table 5-2 Criteria for Including Items in the Annotated Bibliography

1. Published between January 1975 and December 2000

2. Published in one of the peer-reviewed journals listed in Table 5-1

3. Published in an occupational therapy textbook by a reputable commercial publisher

4. Identified consensually by three authors as an occupational conceptual model, according to definitions found in Chapter 2

5. Judged by three authors to have made a significant contribution to the development of occupational therapy theory over the 25-year period

6. Consensually classifiable in one of the five theory areas or as general theory about occupation

7. Indexed with one of the following electronic search mechanisms: OTDBase, Medline, or CINAHL

tual tools that help to explain or predict a central construct or that promote the understanding of a central phenomenon—in our case, occupation.

In the emerging discipline of occupational therapy, many important ideas and concepts are found throughout the literature but not incorporated into well-developed theories or networks of concepts and relationships that would allow explanation or prediction. Yet, these ideas can be most helpful to occupational therapists, students, educators, and researchers to better understand and apply occupation. For our purposes, we include all of these in the present volume.

Further, it should be emphasized that where well-defined theories do exist (we referred to them earlier as *named theories* or *large-T theories*), they may not be able to be neatly classified into one particular slot in the classification system. After all, theory in occupational therapy seldom focuses on one component of occupation. Instead, the classification system offers a way of examining particular ideas or principles within a theory, thus determining their ideological and conceptual origins. To expand the example used in Chapter 3, our classification system considers roles and habits to be socio-cultural determinants of occupation. Therefore, by consulting the socio-cultural section of this book (Chapter 12), we can not only find out how the Model of Human Occupation contributes to our understanding of the social and cultural determinants of occupation, but we can also discover what other theorists have said about roles and habits. However, we cannot assume that because roles and habits are part of the Model of Human Occupation that the whole model is classified as socio-cultural. Other ideas from the model, such as general systems theory (environmental, Chapter 13) or personal causation (psychological-emotional, Chapter 10) belong elsewhere in the classification system. Thus, the taxonomy aims to classify particular ideas that guide understanding and therapeutic action.

In our efforts to be comprehensive in capturing all occupational therapy ideology, we have not restricted our selections by level of theory development or sophistication. We acknowledge that within this volume there exists a wide variety of types and levels of theory. Some of the theoretical material catalogued is sketchy and conditional, whereas other material is well-developed and widely recognized. Readers are cautioned to read this book with the same level of analysis required of all professional reading and to evaluate the concepts presented on the basis of some set of criteria for validity.

Guide for Evaluating Theory

Here are some guidelines for evaluating theory. Readers may wish to consider both internal and external criteria when evaluating theory. Internal criteria refer to those that can be assessed within the article or book in which the theory is found. External criteria are those for which the reader needs to seek additional information beyond the article to evaluate theory. Table 5-3 summarizes internal and external criteria for evaluating theory.

INTERNAL CRITERIA

1. *Uniqueness:* Does the article or book address a unique new way of understanding the phenomenon of interest? Are the ideas contained original, or do they repeat or re-interpret original ideas expressed elsewhere?

2. *Consistency:* Are the relationships and linkages suggested consistent with values, assumptions, and other principles in the model? Does the theoretical idea contain any contradictions or logical inconsistencies? Sometimes it helps to try and diagram the relationships proposed in order to test consistency. If you cannot construct a clear and consistent diagram showing the relationships between concepts proposed in the theory, then perhaps it is because information is either missing or internally inconsistent.

Table 5-3	Criteria for Evaluating Theory

INTERNAL CRITERIA

I	Uniqueness	Does it express a unique and original idea?
2.	Consistency	Are the ideas internally consistent?
3.	Generalizability	Does it have broad or specific applicability?
4.	Utility	Can the ideas be translated into practice?

EXTERNAL CRITERIA

I.	Origins	Are the theoretical/ideological origins apparent?
2.	Source	Where is it published? Is it a reputable source?
3.	Authorship	Are the authors appropriately qualified?

For example, it would be inappropriate in a model of the environmental impacts on occupational therapy to include a detailed analysis of the individual and his or her performance components. The environmental approach locates the problem outside the individual in the environment, therefore, according to this approach, it would be inconsistent to analyse the individual in detail other than to assess where particular environmental components might have an impact.

3. *Utility*: Is it clear how the idea or concept will be used? Does it have understandable implications for practice? Is there a relationship between ideas in the conceptual model and ideas in the model of practice? As discussed in Chapter 2, is it possible to anticipate what the assessments and intervention approaches associated with the model of practice might be?

4. *Generalizability*: Can the ideas be applied broadly to all aspects of occupation and to all possible problems with occupation, or are they specifically intended to help with particular types of people or particular occupational problems?

EXTERNAL CRITERIA

1. *Origins*: What are the ideological origins of the theory or idea being discussed in a particular article or book? Does the author refer to a sound background of basic theory in which the current work is grounded, or is it presented as though it were an entirely new idea? Hopefully, without sounding too cynical, there are relatively few new ideas under the sun. Most good theory is an extension or development of existing theory. For example, we consider object relations theory to be in the domain of occupational conceptual models. Yet, while it is capable of standing on its own merits, the credibility of object relations theory is considerably enhanced by tracing its origins to its psychodynamic and psychoanalytic roots. The author writing about object relations theory today would risk almost certain dismissal if he or she did not demonstrate a familiarity with the history and critique of psychoanalytic theory, and show how his or her new idea overcame previous theoretical or ideological problems.

2. *Source:* Where was the theory published? There is clearly a pecking order of credibility and prestige associated with the source of a publication. We will consider three sources, although there may be many more, including books,refereed journals, and professional publications. To have a commercial book publisher assess your work as unique and marketable is a very credible sign indeed. Book publication involves two elements of credibility: market review and peer review. Market review shows whether or not your theory is unique and whether others are likely be interested enough to buy it. Peer review shows whether or not your work can stand up to the scrutiny of other experts in your field. It means that a panel of experts has reviewed your work to assess whether it meets the professional standard for publication. Journal articles are also subject to peer review. Before an article is published in a refereed journal, two or three experts in the field typically see it, and their comments and suggestions for improvement must be incorporated before it can be published. As a result, a standard of credibility in the professional literature is upheld. There is another type of professional publication, however, that is not peer-reviewed—the practice magazine or newsletter. The articles in these magazines are intended to address practice issues with some immediacy, and, therefore, are not subject to the lengthy process of peer review. That is not to say that they are not credible, only that they have not been subjected to the same level of scrutiny and processing that refereed publications have. There is, of course, a fourth venue for publication that we have not considered yet—the Internet. It is especially important when downloading theoretical information from the Internet to understand the conditions under which it was published. There are numerous reasons why someone would elect to publish theory on the Internet, and the message to the reader is "buyer beware." While there is plenty of good information on the Internet, the reader can be offered no assurances of its quality.

3. *Authorship:* Who is the theorist, and is he or she adequately prepared to be expounding this theory? For the most part, if you look at the theory that comes most readily to mind, the authors are academics and educators. The reason for this is that academics and educators typically work in the world of ideas—this is their stock and trade. That is not to say that they do not understand practice, nor is it to say that practitioners do not understand ideas. It is simply to state the obvious fact that people who work with ideas are more likely to be the producers of ideas, and furthermore, that they are more likely to have access to the time, skills, and means to publish their ideas. Thus, in evaluating theory, particularly conceptual models, we have to ask if the author has the credentials and the systemic or institutional supports to be producing credible theory. Are they associated with others working in the same field? Are they working alone or with collaborators who supplement each others' skill and knowledge sets? For example, when we see theory involving occupational science coming out of the University of Southern California, we make a fairly safe assumption that this work had the benefit of input from the originators of this field of inquiry and that it was probably well-supported in the institutional structure there.

On the other hand, when evaluating a model of practice, credibility is enhanced when authorship includes individuals actually involved in practice. Since models of practice translate conceptual models into the tools for practice (i.e., assessment and intervention approaches), then a model of practice would typically be evaluated more highly if it was developed in consultation with practitioners or practice settings. For example, when Kielhofner began to develop tools for practice (particularly assessments) that expressed the ideas of the Model of Human Occupation, he tended to collaborate with people directly involved in various areas of mental health practice, thereby enhancing both the credibility and the acceptability of these tools.

Summary of the Contents and Organization of the Book

In our evolving discipline, many theories are yet to be developed and expounded by occupational therapists. The present book will hopefully serve not only as a catalogue of theory already developed over the last quarter of the 20th century, but also as a catalyst to theory development in the coming years.

One distinction is important, however. This book does not deal with basic theory or with models of practice (quadrants 2 through 4 of the toolbox). Rather, it focuses on theory that helps us to understand the notion of occupation, the parameters and determinants of occupation, and its centrality for health. The works included in this book are those descriptive or empirical articles that define and analyze occupation (quadrant 1 of the toolbox, occupational conceptual models).

In summary, the present volume began with three basic ideas about occupation: that it is essential to human beings, that it can change, and that it can be used as a therapeutic medium. The first of these ideas was expounded in Chapter 1, and an explicit, generic definition of occupation was offered (see Figure 1-1). In Chapters 2 through 4, two metaphors were offered to help readers think about occupational therapy theory:

- ✖ The toolbox, for sorting and storing the four ways occupational therapists use theory

- ✖ The filing cabinet, for organizing what we know about occupation, to correspond to the generic model in Figure 1-1 (i.e., to correspond to the five known determinants of occupation)

Next, in Chapters 6 and 7, we trace the development of the concept of occupation over the past century, with particular emphasis on the past 25 years. Chapter 8 develops the second basic idea with which the book began, that occupation changes, and Chapter 14 develops the third of these basic ideas, that occupation can be used therapeutically. Chapters 9 through 13 offer annotated bibliographies of conceptual models in occupational therapy. These five chapters correspond to the five determinants of occupation in the generic model of occupation shown in Figure 1-1, to the drawers of the filing cabinet in Figure 3-1, and to the headings of the occupational therapy theory taxonomy in Figure 3-2. Specifically, the five categories of occupational therapy theory are physical determinants of occupation (Chapter 9), psychological-emotional determinants of occupation (Chapter 10), cognitive-neurological determinants of occupation (Chapter 11), socio-cultural determinants of occupation (Chapter 12), and environmental determinants of occupation (Chapter 13).

6 THE CONCEPT OF OCCUPATION 1900 TO 1974

Penny Bryden, PhD and Mary Ann McColl, PhD

This chapter reviews the evolution of the concept of occupation over the first part of the 20th century. Long before the profession of occupational therapy was conceived, the word occupation was used colloquially in much the same way that occupational therapists now use it—to refer to a meaningful way to use time. Jane Austen gives us evidence of this in the novel, *Sense and Sensibility*, when a distraught Col. Brandon says to Eleanor, "Give me some occupation, or I shall run mad!" This, along with popular maxims like "Idle hands are the devil's playground," tells us that not only the concept of occupation, but its health-promoting effects, were common knowledge at the beginning of this century, when occupational therapy came into being. It is therefore only a short step to the definition of occupation advanced by the founders, such as Adolph Meyer (1922): "...a freer conception of work, including recreation and any form of helpful enjoyment."

This holistic view of occupation was soon challenged as the Cartesian mind-body dichotomy pervaded popular culture. It then became important for health professionals to locate problems in either the mind or the body and to differentiate between interventions that were aimed at mind problems from those aimed at body problems. This coupled with the intellectual pressure of the scientific revolution in the 1950s and 60s, and soon the concept of occupation had disappeared from the collective professional radar screen.

In 1962, Reilly refocused the attention of occupational therapists on the health-giving potential of occupation in her Eleanor Clark-Slagle lecture entitled, "Occupational Therapy Can Be One of the Great Ideas of 20th Century Medicine." Gender-specific language notwithstanding, the following quote stands out as a pivotal point in the history of the concept of occupation in occupational therapy: "...Man, through the use of his hands, as they are energized by his mind and will, can influence the state of his own health" (p. 1).

This moment in time represents the beginning of a movement away from the tendency to try to reduce occupation to component parts and to focus treatment on smaller and smaller pieces of human beings. At the same time, it represents a movement toward a rediscovery of the therapeutic power of occupation for individuals, families, communities, and even society.

This chapter offers an overview of occupational therapy theory development over the period from 1900 to 1975, decade by decade. In addition to encapsulating significant events in the theoretical development of occupational therapy, the chapter attempts to place these developments in the context of medical and societal developments.

1900 to 1910

> *How does occupation effect a cure?…One thing is certain, that the coated tongue, the obstinate constipation, the diminished secretions, the sallow complexion and the other symptoms of ill health that very stubbornly resist other methods of treatment gradually disappear when patients are engaged in suitable occupation, and we can nearly always look forward with confidence for a marked improvement in mental condition.*
>
> Moher, T. J. (1907). Occupation in the treatment of the insane.
> JAMA, 158, 1666

> *In these cases in which the tired mind tortures itself with doubts and fears and spends the long days in useless self-analysis, and in appreciation of mental and physical suffering, it is probable that progress toward health is often indefinitely delayed because no occupation is found or ever attempted… A division of the twenty-four hours into changeable periods of work, rest and recreation, plenty of air, wholesome food, wise suggestions and such medical treatment as may be indicated—these simple elements, together with a pretty complete detachment from all other obligations in life, represent in brief the industrial system of treatment."*
>
> Hall, H. J. (1910). Work-cure: A report of 5 years experience at an institution
> devoted to the therapeutic application of manual work.
> JAMA, 55, 12-13

North America embraced the 20th century with a sense of optimism, trusting that the New World had finally come of age. The ideal of a North American utopia gave purpose to a number of reform movements aimed at the development of social welfare services and industrial standards. Humanism was the dominant ideology, and women played an important role in social reform, in addition to struggling for political equality for themselves. In the interest of women's rights, the first day-care centres were established, women sought representation in industrial unions and a balanced routine, including physical activity, came to be increasingly valued. The advent of x-ray technology, blood transfusions, and early anaesthetics allowed dramatic advances in surgical techniques and procedures. These changes in knowledge and technology in the early 20th century brought about a positive shift in the valuing of health care professionals. Medicine began to be associated with science and technology, in place of its historical association with charity. The reform impulse in the health care field aimed toward more effective and efficient treatment of the ill, thus ensuring the continuation of a progressive march toward the future. The predominant diagnoses that figure in the literature of the first decade of this century are a variety of mental and nervous disorders and tuberculosis.

The humanitarian movement of this period contrasted sharply with the intolerance of weakness and abnormality seen in the late 19th century, associated with Darwinism and the notion of survival of the fittest. The early 20th century saw a renaissance of the moral treatment ideals of respect, kindness, religious attendance, daily routines, and diversion from morbid thoughts through labour. Physicians began to express the idea that people were healthier if they were meaningfully occupied. In fact, physicians took a sponsorship role in encouraging nurses and other health attendants to be aware of this idea and to put it into practice. They felt that the presence of occupation, or something to meaningfully occupy one's time, was the key to being healthy. Further, they suggested that one who was busy had no time to dwell on unhealthy notions or practices. Whereas in years gone by, a rest-cure had been a common prescription for ailments of a variety of types, physicians were beginning to talk about a work-cure. They were beginning to prescribe a balanced regimen of work, supervised by a new breed of health workers called occupational therapists.

1910 to 1919

The benefits (of occupational therapy) are (1) The employment of a large number of patients... which causes them to be less introspective; (2) the breaking up of a day full of monotony from which all hope and ambition is removed, into one which for several hours at least the individual has some real reason for existence; (3) the re-education of patients and the training of habits which will permit them to go out into the world and lead a more or less self-sustaining life.

Ricksher, C. (1913). Occupation in the treatment of the insane.
Illinois Medical Journal, 23, 385

At first the benefit of occupation was supposed to be in its time-killing characteristics. In certain advanced and chronic cases, this is all it can be claimed for. In other cases, however, in which there is hope of partial, if not complete, recovery, occupation is found to have certain definite effects. It centres the patient's attention away from himself. Thus mental debris is cleared away, and the real physical symptoms remain, which form a reliable index to the physician in diagnosis and prognosis. The effect of manual work is to strengthen muscles and coordinate the body. Change of occupation stimulates the brain, while continued occupation concentrates it.

Upham, E. G. (1917). Some principles of occupational therapy.
Modern Hospital, 8, 409

World War I dominated the second decade of the 20th century, and the idealism of earlier years was dealt a crushing blow. The reform impulse that characterized the first decade gave way to the need for efficiency and productivity in a tight war-time economy. It came to be believed that any given process, including the treatment of the ill, could be more effectively conducted if different specialists were responsible for each individual task. Science, efficiency, and progress were seen as inextricably linked.

Health care practitioners saw their roles greatly enhanced as the public became increasingly enamoured of all things scientific. War-time casualties brought a focus and legitimacy to physical disability that was previously unknown. As well, automation, industrialization, and the automobile brought with them industrial and vehicular accidents that often result-ed in injury and disability. The polio epidemic of 1916 was another significant feature of this decade that focused the attention of the medical community on individuals with residual physical incapacities and paved the way for the development of the field of rehabilitation. In occupational therapy, the literature of this decade was dominated by a concern for return-ing veterans of the war and for their continued productivity, participation, and dignity. Whereas previously occupation had been applied primarily to mental disorders, its applica-tion for disabled veterans was readily apparent.

At the same time, the fundamental idea of occupation continued to be developed. Articles were devoted to determining the parameters of occupation and the principles for choosing and prescribing occupation relative to a specific problem. For example, occupation was felt to be most therapeutic if it was suited to the individual and, therefore, motivating and interesting. Further, the notion of productivity was explored, both from the perspective of a tangible end product, as well as from the perspective of economic viability. The idea was introduced of preparing individuals for future remunerative work and of matching the individual's capabilities and interests to therapeutic activities. The importance of graded activity, or activity that could be adapted so that it continuously provided a challenge, was examined. In 1920, the first mention is made of occupational therapy with a child.

1920 to 1929

We know we are helping these misfit children to self-possession in the broadest sense of the word, to realize that they are responsible little folks with real things to do. We help them to form good habits, to be observant, attentive, cooperative, honest, well-behaved children. We know that their salvation lies in handwork, and so we are encouraged to try again and again…

Bryant, L. C. (1926). Manual work with the mentally defective child patient. *Modern Hospital, 27,* 63

But occupational therapy has a very definite place, and it may be as a leading American psychiatrist of international reputation has said, "occupational therapy will some day rank with anaesthetics in taking the suffering out of sickness."

Walker, J. (1920). Occupational therapy. *Occupational Therapy and Rehabilitation, 9,* 201

The decade known as the "roaring twenties" was initially characterized by two significant movements: women's suffrage and prohibition. Women's groups were able to use their con-tribution to the war effort to promote their right to vote. By the early 1920s, most North American women had gained the right to vote, and the prohibition lobby attempted to cap-italize on the austerity of the war years. It was not until later in the 1920s that North Americans began to experience the seemingly limitless optimism that usually characterizes popular accounts of the time. Industries began to respond to the developments in technol-ogy, and consumers responded to the abundance of goods on the market. The result was an artificially high level of prosperity. Automobiles, telephones, and radios freed up large amounts of time, and people began to look for ways to spend their newfound leisure time. The collapse of the stock market in 1929 was an almost predictable response to the euphoric climate of investment and to the overextension of credit.

In the medical arena, the most significant advance of this decade was the popular acceptance of the "germ theory" of disease etiology, and the corresponding development of vaccines and public health measures. Epidemics of communicable diseases, such as typhoid and small pox, were virtually eliminated, making way for a focus on illnesses of a more chronic nature. Women played a vital role in educating the poor on the importance of personal and public hygiene, as well as serving as primary care givers in the recuperative process. Public hospitals flourished, and medicine became increasingly associated with the sciences. The biomedical model emerged, with its roots in utilitarianism, science, and rationality. It emphasized the importance of accurate diagnoses, using the most advanced technologies, and the application of scientifically sound treatments to cure pathology in the body and mind. In the mental health field, two other major schools of thought were emerging. The works of Freud and the psychoanalytic theorists, and Pavlov and the behaviourists led to a view of mental illness as psychologically determined, rather than physiologically or structurally caused.

Occupational therapy services in chronic institutions expanded greatly during the 1920s, to the point where few were without occupational therapists. In addition, the discipline undertook a number of maintenance tasks, such as the development of professional associations, a journal, and educational standards. Occupational therapy was defined in this decade as "any activity, mental or physical, definitely prescribed and guided for the distinct purpose of contributing to and hastening recovery from disease or injury" (Pattison, 1922). The literature still emphasized the use of graded, goal-oriented activity to motivate the patient toward recovery; and the balance of work, rest, and play in a person's daily occupations were considered vital to recovery. Seminal publications by Adolph Meyer and Eleanor Clarke-Slagle advanced the basic ideas underlying occupational therapy for this period: the idea of a balance of work, rest, and play for health and the importance of regular, purposeful activity to organize one's time and roles.

In the last 5 years of this decade, the increasing influence of the medical profession and the emerging biomedical model can be observed in the occupational therapy literature of the day. Some examples of these trends include the reference to the body as a physical machine, the need for basic science in occupational therapy curricula, references to occupational therapy as a medical, not a social, field, and the increasing emphasis on return to work rather than the holistic curative aspects of occupation. The first reference to physical rehabilitation and to matching the activity to the disease (as well as to the person) appears in this decade.

A debate also began to emerge about the economic aspects of therapy. Was therapy primarily curative or should the products of therapy be economically useful and marketable? The works of Karl Marx brought new sensitivity to the issues of exploitation of workers, which had implications for the field of industrial therapy. In an effort to ensure that patients were not abused, some institutions shifted from involving patients in the actual work of the institution to simulated work, particularly crafts.

1930 to 1939

The decade of the 1930s was dominated by the Great Depression. Although predictable in hindsight, it took North America almost entirely by surprise. Business collapse alone would have made life difficult enough for North Americans in the decade of the 1930s, but

> *Modern society is organized on an occupational basis, it is the occupation of the individual which gives him a feeling of independence and at the same time binds him to society.*
>
> Le Vesconte, H. P. (1934). The place of occupational therapy in social work planning. *Canadian Journal of Occupational Therapy 2,* 13
>
> *...A dementia praecox can play baseball, while a dementia paralytica can bowl.*
>
> Losada, C. A. (1936). Some values in occupational therapy. *Occupational Therapy and Rehabilitation, 15,* 288

combined with drought, thousands were left destitute. Relief programs ranging from agricultural support to job creation in industry and public works did not end the depression, but at least they offered new ways of surviving it. This era marked the beginning of a more active role for government in the lives of individuals. However, the enclave of medicine remained relatively impervious to government intervention, despite calls for national health insurance to care for the illness and poverty caused by the depression.

The expansion of occupational therapy services was dramatically halted over the decade of the 1930s. Although occupational therapy often contributed positively to the economics of a hospital by hastening recovery and discharge, many occupational therapy departments were reduced or closed. An appeal was made for therapists to continue their good works on a voluntary basis, harkening back to a time when all female labor was considered philanthropic. Occupational therapy, however, was striving to be recognized as a legitimate discipline within the medical care system and spurned these entreaties toward voluntarism. It was during this period that the debate began over diversionary versus therapeutic activity, and one of the original tenets of occupational therapy—that diversionary activity was therapeutic—was temporarily lost.

The literature in this decade shows little real ideological growth, as occupational therapy, along with society in general, was preoccupied with survival. Articles continued to reflect occupational therapy's commitment to the use of purposeful, productive activity to promote social and economic adjustment, and the debate over the need to produce articles of economic value in occupational therapy continued. Evidence abounds for the increasing influence of the biomedical model. Concepts of activity analysis and graduated exercise were central to the literature of this decade. Whereas several decades earlier occupational therapy had dealt almost exclusively with mental health, by 1937, the tables had turned to the point where Clarke (1937) suggested that occupational therapy should expand beyond physical activities into the psychosocial field!

1940 to 1949

With the memories of World War I still fresh in many of their minds, North Americans embarked on another "war to end all wars." Men and women from both Canada and the United States were quick to respond to the call to arms and also to financially support the Allied war effort. On the home front, the last vestiges of the depression vanished as industries sprang to work putting out war supplies. Women played a dominant role in factories, as well as on the farms, filling in for men who were fighting overseas.

> *Civilization itself may indeed be defined to some extent as the ability of mankind to adjust itself to its handicaps by the successful application of the various modalities of occupational therapy and its related specialties… When psychotherapy is crossed with physical therapy, we have occupational therapy, with the best characteristics of both parent specialties.*
>
> Bluestone, E. M. (1942). The argument for occupational therapy. *Occupational Therapy and Rehabilitation, 21,* 222
>
> *When the choice of activity was removed from the whims of the patient to the considered thought of the therapist, occupational therapy gained scientific status.*
>
> Licht, S., & Reilly, M. (1943). The correlation of physical and occupational therapy. *Occupational Therapy and Rehabilitaion, 22,* 171

The experience of war had served to revive interest in health insurance and social security to combat the contingencies of unemployment, old age, and ill health. Preliminary discussions took place about the development of health insurance, but no real policy action was to take place until long after the war had ended.

In the medical field, a number of crucial developments during this decade changed the face of medical practice and rehabilitation. First, the discovery of penicillin and antibiotics put a virtual end to many communicable disease epidemics by 1950, making way for an increase in the prevalence of chronic conditions. Second, medical and surgical improvements during the war led to the survival of casualties who would formerly have died of infection or other traumatic complications. Both of these developments required a tangible response from the medical profession and the emerging rehabilitation professions because of the increased prevalence of disability in society. In the mental health field, the advent of neuroleptic drugs and electroconvulsive therapy during the 1940s dramatically altered the practice of psychiatry. Instead of physical restraints, drugs rendered formerly unmanageable patients docile and amenable to psychological therapies.

Occupational therapists responded to these developments with formal techniques and programs of activities of daily living, vocational and prevocational assessment, and training. These domains of occupation (i.e., self-care, leisure, and work) came to be regarded as separate domains, rather than as elements of an integrated and balanced occupational whole. Developments of synthetic materials for industry crossed over to the medical field to permit advances in prosthetic and orthotic technology. Again, occupational therapists responded with techniques to promote skill and expertise in their patients with these new devices in much the same way that they sought skill and expertise in their own professional domain.

1950 to 1959

The decade of the 1950s was marked by the Cold War on the international front, and by a buoyant economy on the home front. Business and industry flourished in a climate of almost insatiable demand for products of every description, from homes to cars to appliances to clothes. This era of plenty not only encouraged a dramatic rise in domestic population (the "baby boom"), but also lured hundreds of thousands of immigrants from war-torn European and Asian countries.

> *Occupational therapy, born as a war baby during World War I, has had many years to mature, yet the question arises whether she has come of age. She often serves as one of the handmaidens of medicine; at other times she works alone without any seeming relationship to the great family of medicine. Some workers in the medical field question whether she is indeed a true member of the family.*
>
> Gordon, E. E. (1954). Does occupational therapy meet the demands of total rehabilitation? *Am J Occup Ther, 8,* 238

> *... Integrated function is the keynote. For this reason, the use of simple, normal, life-like activities is a logical treatment to encourage response in paresis in muscles. This, of course, is a principle of occupational therapy. Then occupational therapy should inherently, by the nature of its approach, be helpful in these cases.*
>
> Ayres, A. J. (1955). Proprioceptive facilitation elicited through the upper extremities. *Am J Occup Ther, 9,* 121

> *In occupational therapy, the activities which you are going to do need to be done over and over and over, and they have to be fun, and they have to be done properly. We haven't done what we need to do in occupational therapy. We need to study. We need an understanding just as we need our basic science.*
>
> Rood, M. (1956). Neurophysiological mechanisms utilized in the treatment of neuromuscular dysfunction. *Am J Occup Ther, 10,* 224

The 1950s were also a time of technological and scientific innovations. The exigencies of war and the continued participation in the Cold War had ramifications for advances in both the areas of space technology and medicine. While aeronautical engineers discovered new ways to broaden the world's horizons, medical researchers opened new frontiers in the treatment of illness. Pharmacological advances brought about a mentality that virtually every disorder could be treated with drugs, and physicians lost no time in prescribing new medications for mental and physical illness. Penicillin, the wonder drug of the last decade, became widely used in the 1950s, and the discovery of the polio vaccine mid-decade meant that polio was virtually eliminated, although many survivors experienced residual disabilities. In the newly recognized field of rehabilitation, territorial disputes were underway as the team concept developed. Instead of promoting cooperation and integration, the team concept brought pressure to bear on young health disciplines to differentiate themselves, to become increasingly specialized and to claim their area of expertise through research and technology.

Developments in neurological research put information at the disposal of occupational therapists. Consistent with the prevailing biomedical, reductionist philosophy, occupational therapists began to apply this information to address specific physical or skill-related problems, consistent with a general trend to emphasize technique rather than theory.

In the mental health field, dramatic changes were taking place. Theory borrowed from sociology underlined the importance of groups for social interaction and mental health. The group became a focus for therapy and was seen to have therapeutic properties unattainable in individual therapy. Applications of theory from psychology, particularly psychoanalytic theory, increased the awareness of occupational therapists of the power of the unconscious and the therapeutic benefits of unlocking information held at an unconscious level. Projective techniques became part of the arsenal of the occupational therapist, and different approaches were advanced to explore psychodynamic processes. Finally, the increasing sophistication of psychotropic drugs not only led to more freedom for patients in institutions, but also in the community. Former mental patients began to be discharged to the community in unprecedented numbers, to be absorbed by an ill-prepared society.

1960 to 1969

> *The logic of occupational therapy rests upon the principle that man has a need to master his environment, to alter and improve it. When this need is blocked by disease or injury, severe dysfunction and unhappiness result. Man must develop and exercise the powers of his central nervous system through open encounter with life around him. Failure to spend and to use what he has in the performance of the tasks that belong to his role in life makes him less human than he could be.*
>
> Reilly, M. (1962). Occupational therapy can be one of the great ideas of 20th century medicine. *Am J Occup Ther, 16,* 6

> *The social problem which really exists has to do with the treatment of long-term patients... If occupational therapy is to contribute to a reduction of this great social problems it will be necessary for therapists to consider the way they approach treatment. They must be concerned with all the activities of living—not techniques but the use of the self in motivating and leading patients towards effective living.*
>
> Roberts, C. A. (1962). Healing the sick—responsibility or privilege—for the patient for the therapist. *Canadian Journal of Occupational Therapy, 29,* 13

The continued economic boom throughout the decade of the 1960s provided the necessary stability for a fundamental re-evaluation of the relationships, responsibilities, and obligations that society had forged. The solutions proposed were often radical, but the realization of inequities was something that no one could ignore. Protest groups fought for civil rights for African Americans, and feminists attacked the hierarchical structure of North American society. In the face of continued pressure, government increased its capacity to function as both mediator and provider.

With Canadian and American governments showing increased concern about social and political rights of citizens, scientific advancements in both countries continued at astonishing speed. Vast sums of money were spent to encourage research and development, particularly in areas that would have an immediate effect on the well-being of the population. The health field especially benefited from this new focus, with important advances being made in techniques for diagnosis and treatment.

In occupational therapy, the speed and extent of change brought about a feeling of collective insecurity about the "complexity of illness relative to the simplicity of our tools" (Reilly, 1962). The pride of the developing profession seen in previous decades was replaced by a sense of doubt and conflict. The professional literature illustrates a response to this crisis through an increasing focus on science, rather than occupation.

1970 to 1974

> *Imagine we occupational therapists are like a child standing on the sidewalk holding a balloon on a string, and watching a big parade of medical and scientific progress go by. Every now and again, like a child, we attempt to join the parade; we try to put on the regalia of professional jargon, but it doesn't fit too well. Despite the paternal amusement of our more sophisticated colleagues in other professions, we have not let go of the string of the balloon—at least, I hope this is true, for in my story, it is a beautiful balloon representing an understanding of the value of human potential.*
>
> Schimeld, A. (1971). Youth of today and their influences on the practice of occupational therapy. *Canadian Journal of Occupational Therapy, 38*, 9
>
> *One of the problems of moving from the medical model to the biopsychosocial model has to do with change itself. Any change is uncomfortable. However it must be remembered that occupational therapists really did not use the medical model for ordering a theoretical base or practice... A realistic problem concerns the professional self-concept: a therapist who uses the biopsychosocial model has a much heavier emphasis upon the teaching-learning process.*
>
> Mosey, A .C. (1974). An alternative: The biopsychosocial model. *Am J Occup Ther, 28*, 140

The relatively stable economies of the 1950s and 60s left North Americans unprepared for the recession of the 1970s. In response, politicians began to seriously question the social and public policy goals of the previous generation in an attempt to come to terms with new realities. Events like the Vietnam War and the Watergate scandal brought about a new period of popular cynicism. More moderate forms of protest replaced radical movements, and both women and people of color made fewer gains. The economic recession predisposed politicians to careful evaluation of resource implications, rather than to action.

However, this spirit of questioning and accountability had notable effects on the health field in general, and occupational therapy in particular. A new emphasis was placed on quality assurance, standards of care, and the development of audit tools and methods. Also connected with the need for accountability is a strong push in the 1970s toward professionalism. The process of professionalization was initially seen as related to the acquisition of the characteristics of true professions, particularly an exclusive body of knowledge. Thus, the literature of the early 1970s is characterized by a preliminary discussion in nearly every article of the need for theory, accountability, and professionalism. This was a period of dramatic developments in the neurosciences, when occupational therapists made the most of an enriched understanding of the neuro-muscular system.

Conclusion

This chapter has summarized the development of occupational therapy theory in the North American context from 1900 to 1974. The next chapter looks in greater detail at the development of the concept of occupation over the period of 1975 to 2000.

References

Clarke, B. (1937). The use of ocucpational therapy in social stabilization: Results of recent research. *Occupational Therapy and Rehabilitation, 16,* 143-58

Meyer A. (1922). The philosophy of occupational therapy. *Archives of Occupational Therapy, 1,* 1-10.

Pattison, H. A. (1922). The trend of occupational therapy for tuberculosis. *Archives of Occupational Therapy, 1,* 19-24.

Reilly, M. (1962). Occupational therapy can be one of the great ideas of 20th century medicine. *Am J Occup Ther, 16,* 1-9.

7

THE CONCEPT OF OCCUPATION 1975 TO 2000

Mary Ann McColl, PhD

The period between 1975 and 2000 saw a renaissance of the concept of occupation as central to occupational therapy. During the last 25 years of the 20th century, occupational therapy theorists sought to refine the definition of occupation, to distinguish it from other related terms, and to develop a knowledge base about occupation that was theoretically consistent and empirically supported. Table 7-1 offers some definitions of occupation that appear in the literature over the past 25 years and illustrate the evolving concept.

The period begins with numerous historical reviews of the profession of occupational therapy, with emphasis on the concept of occupation. Each of these articles summarizes with the same conclusion that occupational therapy must return to its roots and re-establish its professional territory in the area of occupation. By the early 1980s, momentum was established for the development of a science of occupation.

The mid-1980s also saw a focus on the environment as a target for treatment. The impact of the independent living movement had begun to be felt in the profession of occupational therapy. According to the independent living ideology, disability was historically ill-construed as a function of the person, whereas it was at least as much a function of an environment created to conform to an able-bodied bias. Thus, disability came to be seen not simply as an organic reality but also as a socially constructed phenomenon. Coupled with broad societal concern for the impact of the industrialized world on the physical environment, this trend had a significant impact on the field of occupational therapy. The environment was defined, characterized, and conceptualized, alongside the person, as a legitimate source of occupational therapy intervention. Theory from other disciplines, such as systems theory and ecological theory, helped to inform this new approach.

Another notable undertaking of the literature of the 1980s includes attempts to study and understand the nature and characteristics of occupation, both as a naturally occurring phenomenon and as a therapeutic medium. With the development of qualitative research methods in the 1980s and 1990s, occupation came to be understood not simply as an objective, observable phenomenon, but also as an experienced, personal, and subjective phenomenon. Qualitative methods drew occupational therapists into a closer understanding of the unique nature of each person's occupational experience, and the extent to which it was embedded

Table 7-1	The Evolving Definition of Occupation

Mosey (1981)

* Defined the domain of concern of occupational therapy as performance components: sensory, motor, neurological, cognitive, psychological, and social
* These performance components are influenced by age, environment, and occupation

Katz (1985)

* Advocated for reconsideration of the domain of concern of occupational therapy as occupation

Mosey (1985)

* Advocated for a pluralistic view of occupational therapy
* Pluralism defined as acceptance of many basic ideas and principles; occupational therapy defined by numerous elements, each with associated principles
* Monism defined as the governance of reality by a single idea or principle

Kielhofner (1985)

* Advocated for a single unifying idea at the core of occupational therapy (i.e., occupation)

Reed (1986)

* Characterized occupational therapy according to the use of media
* Choices of media governed by a number of factors (cultural, social, political, economic, technological, theoretical, historical, and empirical)

Allen (1987)

* Defined activity as the medium through which humans interact with the environment
* Occupational therapy uses activity, or "bits of life," to overcome problems associated with disability

Nelson (1988)

* Attempted to differentiate parameters of occupation
* Occupational form = context of occupation, circumstances, meaning, and environment
* Occupational performance = objectively observable act of carrying out an occupation

Yerxa (1990)

* As with any mature profession, occupational therapy has an academic discipline underlying practice
* Occupational science = the systematic study of occupation, and the body of knowledge about occupation

Table 7-1 (continued)	The Evolving Definition of Occupation

Mosey (1993)

- ✗ Appealed for a durable connection between the theoretical and applied sciences associated with occupational therapy

Clark (1993)

- ✗ Explored occupation as phenomenology and experience
- ✗ Advocated for narrative as a means of understanding the phenomenological aspect of occupation

Wood (1995)

- ✗ Used weaving as a metaphor for occupational therapy
- ✗ Warp (structure) = engagement in occupation as a therapeutic medium
- ✗ Weft (process) = phenomenology/experience of occupation

Christiansen (1999)

- ✗ Explored occupation as a means of formation and maintenance of identity
- ✗ Introduced idea of personal projects as a way of conceptualizing complex occupations

in context. Numerous articles examined the extent to which particular features of occupation, such as choice, meaning, intensity, and purpose, affected overall outcomes. The nature of engagement in occupation was studied, with a number of articles focusing on the phenomenon of flow, or the altered perceptions that occur when one is optimally engaged in occupation. There was also a renewed interest in crafts as therapeutic media, and a re-examination of the purpose and applications of crafts as occupations.

Yerxa and colleagues from the University of Southern California kicked off the last decade of the 20th century by coining and defining the term *occupational science*, to refer to the scientific discipline associated with the profession of occupational therapy. Considerable discussion ensued about the ability of the profession to support a separate scientific discipline; however, its necessity was understood by all if the field was to advance as required. In addition to guidelines for education and research in the area of occupational science, there were even several attempts at the development of an animal model for the study of human occupation.

Finally, the latter part of the 20th century was marked by a focus on client-centred practice as a basic approach in occupational therapy. This approach is based on beliefs about the dignity and autonomy of human beings and about the nature of therapeutic change. A number of articles and books appear in the last decade, attempting to put this challenging concept into practice.

KEYWORDS USED IN THIS CHAPTER			
Activity	Education	Knowledge	Terminology
Adaptation	Environment	Monism	Therapeutic
Balance	Habit	Models	relationship
Biopsychosocial	Hierarchy	Phenomenology	Time
Competence	History	Philosophy	Values
Development	Humanism	Play	Work
Disability	Identity	Pluralism	

Bibliographic Entries for Occupation (1975 to 2000)

The following annotated bibliography of selected references from journals and books illustrates how these developments took place over time and who were the primary contributors.

1. Engelhardt, H. T. (1977). Defining occupational therapy: The meaning of therapy and the virtues of occupation. *Am J Occup Ther, 31,* 666-672.

Keywords: activity, history, humanism

This article first traces the history of occupation and discusses the importance of activity. Occupational therapy is viewed as having a holistic and humanistic view of health. A model of occupational therapy practice is suggested, which views the profession as a humanistic art. The virtues and burdens of a humanistic approach to therapy are discussed.

2. Meyer, A. (1977). The philosophy of occupational therapy. *Am J Occup Ther, 31,* 639-642.

Keywords: balance, time, philosophy

This is a commemorative reprint of Meyer's seminal 1922 article, in which basic concepts of occupation, balance, and time were defined and expounded.

3. Shannon, P. D. (1977). The derailment of occupational therapy. *Am J Occup Ther, 31,* 229-234.

Keywords: adaptation, competence, values

This article contends that occupational therapy has lost sight of its founding values and beliefs (i.e., has been "derailed"). Shannon recommends a recommitment to the founding philosophy of occupational therapy and the adoption of the occupational behavior paradigm. This paradigm allows occupational therapists to broaden their understanding of the adaptation process as a competency phenomenon.

4. Fidler, G. S., & Fidler, J. W. (1978). Doing and becoming: Purposeful action and self-actualization. *Am J Occup Ther, 32,* 305-310.

Keywords: activity, identity

This paper reviews theoretical constructs in social and individual psychology that provide perspectives for understanding human action. It defines doing as "purposeful action that enables the nascent human to become humanized." It views doing as the basis for physical, mental, and social development, and is essential for competence and adaptation. The article ends with a prescription for doing.

5. Kielhofner, G., & Burke, J. (1980). A model of human occupation. Part 1. Conceptual framework and content. *Am J Occup Ther, 34,* 572-581.

Keywords: essence, systems

This article is the first in a series of four that presents a model of human occupation. It describes humans as occupational creatures. Concepts borrowed from general systems theory are used to build the structural framework of input, throughput, output, and feedback. The interaction between a living system and the environment is stressed.

6. Mosey, A. C. (1980). A model for occupational therapy in mental health. *Occupational Therapy in Mental Health, 1,* 11-31.

Keyword: biopsychosocial

In this article, a model for occupational therapy is presented that is an elaboration of the biopsychosocial model. The model identifies philosophical assumptions, ethical code, filters for selecting theoretical data, theoretical foundation, domain of concern, principles for sequencing practice, and legitimate tools for occupational therapy. The model is intended to give unity to the various frames of reference of the profession.

7. Reed, K. L., & Sanderson, S. R. (1980). *Concepts of occupational therapy.* Baltimore: Williams & Wilkins.

Keywords: knowledge, values

This is one of the first of a new wave of textbooks aimed at outlining the values, processes, and knowledge base of occupational therapy, all based on the concept of occupation. Reed and Sanderson define occupation in terms of self-maintenance, productivity, and leisure.

8. Yerxa, E.J. (1980). Occupational therapy's role in creating a future climate of caring. *Am J Occup Ther, 34,* 529-534.

Keywords: activity, humanism, science

The author examines current trends in society that have influenced the practice and philosophy of occupational therapy. The challenge for the future is to preserve and enhance a climate of caring for patients in the face of a society increasingly dominated by technique and objectivism. This can be done by promoting a new view of health based on occupation rather than on pathology, and by revitalizing the use of arts and crafts, play, work, and self-maintenance skills. The concluding recommendation is that occupational therapists need to identify and define the unique science of human occupation.

9. Bing, R. K. (1981). Occupational therapy revisited: A paraphrastic journey. *Am J Occup Ther, 35,* 499-518.

Keywords: history, humanism, values

A comprehensive historical review of occupational therapy is the focus of this lecture. Through an examination of occupational therapy's ancestral roots, the author specifies several lessons that occupational therapists can learn: the belief in the wholeness of the human—that the mind and body are conjoined, the science fundamental to occupational therapy practice is the natural science of the human, occupational therapy is the only major health profession that focuses on the total human organism's involvement in tasks, any differentiation between occupational therapy and other health providers must have as its major theme occupation and leisure, occupational therapists must continue to strive on behalf of those who are not highly valued by society, and the legacy of experience should be passed on and applied to our present practice.

10. Bissell, J. C., & Mailloux, Z. (1981). The use of crafts in occupational therapy for the physically disabled. *Am J Occup Ther, 35,* 369-374.

Keywords: activity, history

The historical use of crafts in occupational therapy for physical disabilities is reviewed, along with the results of a survey aimed at describing current craft use. The results of the survey showed that therapists are using techniques not unique to occupational therapy and very few therapeutic craft activities. Therapists appeared to stress the physical aspects of therapy with less emphasis on psychosocial and social concerns. Suggestions for the future practice of occupational therapy include the use of therapeutic crafts.

11. Fidler, G. S. (1981). From crafts to competence. *Am J Occup Ther, 35,* 567-573.

Keywords: activity, competence, history

This paper begins with a review of occupational therapy literature to identify the focus and concerns of the profession. The historical view of crafts is outlined, including the evolving relationship between purposeful activities and the sense of competence. It is recommended that the concept of competence in occupational therapy be further explored.

12. Johnson, J. (1981). Old values – new directions: Competence, adaptation, integration. *Am J Occup Ther, 35,* 589-598.

Keywords: humanism, science, values

The current conflict of occupational therapists is explored: that is, the conflict between old values of humanism and caring and the new values and directions of science, objectivity, and dehumanization. The evolution of occupational therapy in the professional literature is reviewed. The author concludes that we can merge old and new values, thereby strengthening each. Traditional values, when supplemented and supported by new knowledge, offer occupational therapists the potential to provide a resource that enables individuals to live their lives as they want and to become what they want to be.

13. Mosey, A. C. (1981). *Occupational therapy: Configurations of a profession.* New York: Raven Press.

Keywords: biopsychosocial, knowledge, values

In this book, Mosey outlines the characteristics of a profession, including a philosophical base, ethical code, theoretical base, domain of concern, principles guiding practice, and legitimate tools. She defines each of these for occupational therapy. The book develops and extends the biopsychosocial model, proposed in 1974, which focuses on physical, psychological, and social components of the person.

14. Kielhofner, G. (1982). A heritage of activity: Development of theory. *Am J Occup Ther, 36,* 723-730.

Keywords: activity, essence, history

The theoretical and ideological heritage of occupational therapy is explored, and principles are identified that are applicable to today's theory and practice. It is argued that the organizing premise for theory should be the concept of occupation, instead of adaptation, development, or activity. The author concludes that occupational therapists need to develop the premise that occupation is a determinant of health.

15. Kielhofner, G. (1982). Habits and habit dysfunction: A clinical perspective for occupational therapy. *Occupational Therapy in Mental Health, 2,* 1-21.

Keyword: habit

The paper revives the concept of habits from its historical position in occupational therapy. The concept is interpreted within the context of the model of human occupation and is understood in terms of its relationship to meeting environmental needs and volitional expectations. Clinical guidelines for habit formation and modification are presented.

16. Canadian Association of Occupational Therapists. (1983). *Occupational therapy: Guidelines for the client-centred practice.* Toronto, ON: CAOT ACE.

Keywords: knowledge, values

These guidelines were the result of a national consensus process aimed at developing a model of practice for occupational therapy in Canada. They were influential in placing occupation at the centre and representing an official move away from a component-based practice.

17. Hinojosa, J., Sabari, J., & Rosenfeld, M. S. (1983). Purposeful activities. *Am J Occup Ther, 37, 805-806.*

Keywords: activity, competence

This is a position paper clarifying the use of the term *purposeful activities* in occupational therapy. Purposeful activities are used by occupational therapists to achieve competence in self-care, work, and play. They provide feedback to the client and the therapist about the client's performance. Successful performance of purposeful activities promotes feelings of competence and provides opportunities for achievement of mastery of the environment.

18. Licht, S. (1983). The early history of occupational therapy: An outline. *Occupational Therapy in Mental Health, 3, 67-88.*

Keyword: history

This paper outlines the historical development of occupational therapy from the time of the ancient Greeks to World War II. This historical use of music, exercise, and work are outlined, and the naming of the profession as occupational therapy by George Barton is discussed.

19. Breines, E. (1984). An attempt to define purposeful activity. *Am J Occup Ther, 38, 543-544.*

Keywords: activity, environment

The author examines the definition and philosophical origins of *purposeful activity* to assist her in defining roles for occupational therapists. She concludes that purposeful activity must be defined in terms of the individual. It is subject to the influence of the structural and personal environment of the individual. Purposeful activities elicit choice and provoke development. Occupational therapists should emphasize the developmental process rather than the specific tools of treatment.

20. Llorens, L. (1984). Theoretical conceptualizations of occupational therapy: 1960-1982. *Occupational Therapy in Mental Health, 4,* 1-14.

Keywords: history, models

A descriptive chronology of conceptualizations of occupational therapy from 1960 to 1982 is presented. Major theoretical frames of reference and common theory bases underlying occupational therapy practice are identified. Examples of these include developmental theory, sensory integration, the biopsychosocial model, temporal adaptation, neuro-rehabilitation, the model of human occupation, and occupational behaviour. The question of the apparent lack of theoretical conceptualizations of practice based on biomechanical approaches is raised.

21. Llorens, L. (1984). Changing balance: Environment and individual. *Am J Occup Ther, 38,* 29-34.

Keywords: balance, environment

The individual is viewed as the first of three levels of environment that must be balanced in the occupational therapy process. The role of occupational therapy is to change the balance from illness to health, from dysfunction to function, or from passivity to activity. The function of purposeful activity or occupation is to facilitate change in the individual environment.

22. Reed, K. L. (1984). *Models of practice in occupational therapy.* Baltimore: Williams & Wilkins.

Keywords: knowledge, models

This book is a comprehensive survey of knowledge used in occupational therapy. Reed advances a complex taxonomy of different types of models, including meta models, super models, health, rehabilitation, generic, parameter, and descriptive models.

23. Rogers, J. C. (1984). Why study human occupation? *Am J Occup Ther, 38,* 47-49.

Keywords: knowledge, science

The study of human occupation is viewed as critical for occupational therapy. The mission of occupational therapy is defined as applying knowledge of occupation to individuals whose occupational behavior is dysfunctional or at risk. Therapists need to understand the development of occupation, to recognize and comprehend problems in occupational performance, and to restore or enhance health through occupation.

24. **West, W. L. (1984). A reaffirmed philosophy and practice of occupational therapy for the 1980s.** *Am J Occup Ther, 38, 15-23.*

Keywords: history, philosophy, values

A review of occupational therapy literature from 1978 to 1983 is presented, along with futurist literature. The founding belief in occupation should be reaffirmed. Four recommendations are made to help re-root occupational therapy in its earliest philosophical traditions: (1) consistent use of the term *occupation* in its broadest sense, (2) references to serving the occupational needs of clients rather than "treating the whole person," (3) organization around occupational performance dysfunction rather than disabilities, and (4) renewal of the commitment to mind-body-environment relationships activated through occupation.

25. **Harvey-Krefting, L. (1985). The concept of work in occupational therapy: A historical review.** *Am J Occup Ther, 39, 301-307.*

Keywords: history, work

Through review of the literature, the author shows that work has been a central part of occupational therapy's unique contribution to the health care field. Despite many changes in the philosophy and theoretical approaches, the focus on work has remained. The conceptual definitions and therapeutic uses of work are described in four developmental stages throughout the history of occupational therapy. The need for work to continue to be central to our profession and to be redefined as history evolves is the concluding recommendation.

26. **Katz, N. (1985). Occupational therapy domain of concern reconsidered.** *Am J Occup Ther, 39, 518-524.*

Keywords: biopsychosocial, monism

The purpose of this article is to reanalyse Mosey's conceptualization of the domain of concern for occupational therapy, as written in her book *Occupational Therapy: Configuration of a Profession* (1981). The author differs from Mosey on two points: (1) the domain of concern should be human occupation instead of performance components, and (2) two additional parameters of occupation should be considered: time and the cultural environment.

27. **Kielhofner, G. (1985). *A model of human occupation: Theory and applications*. Baltimore: Williams & Wilkins.**

Keywords: models, systems

This book advances Kielhofner's model of human occupation. The model represents a systems approach in which occupation is the output and the person is the throughput, conceived as a heirarchy of volitional, habituation, and performance subsystems.

28. Kielhofner, G. (1985). The demise of diffidence: An agenda for occupational therapy. *Canadian Journal of Occupational Therapy, 52,* 165-171.

Keywords: knowledge, monism, philosophy

This article outlines a strategy to bring about the demise of diffidence in occupational therapy. The strategy is laid out relative to three areas: clinical practice, theoretical empirical validation, and philosophical foundations. Recommendations for action on the part of individual therapists and occupational therapy associations are identified. At the heart of this strategy is a focus on occupation as the unifying concept in occupational therapy.

29. Mosey, A. C. (1985). A monistic or pluralistic approach to professional identity? *Am J Occup Ther, 39,* 504-509.

Keywords: pluralism, philosophy

This article describes two approaches that a profession can take in articulating its identity: monistic and pluralistic. A monistic approach states that there is one basic principle that defines a profession. Pluralism is the belief that a number of elements make up a profession, each of which is distinct for its contribution. Mosey advocates for a pluralistic professional identity for occupational therapy.

30. Serrett, K., Newbury, S., Tabacco, A., & Trimble, J. (1985). Adolf Meyer: Contributions to the conceptual foundation of occupational therapy. *Occupational Therapy in Mental Health, 5,* 69-75.

Keywords: biopsychosocial, philosophy, systems

In October of 1921, Meyer presented his fundamental thinking on occupational therapy at the Fifth Annual Meeting of the National Society for the Promotion of Occupational Therapy in his classic paper, "Philosophy of Occupational Therapy." This article is a collection of quotes dealing with such diverse topics as systems theory, holistic treatment, and occupation as a necessary component of life and psychobiology.

31. Kielhofner, G. (1986). Organization of knowledge in occupational therapy: A proposal and survey of the literature. *Occupational Therapy Journal of Research, 6,* 67-84.

Keywords: knowledge, models

This article reviews two existing proposals for organizing knowledge in occupational therapy, asserting the importance of taxonomy for developing epistemology. The author proposes a modified approach that synthesizes features of both and then classifies the contents of one prominent occupational therapy journal over a 10-year period to test the utility of the model and to reveal trends in the body of knowledge.

32. Reed, K. (1986). Tools of practice: Heritage or baggage? *Am J Occup Ther, 40,* 597-605.

Keywords: activity, work

This article discusses the major factors that influence the selection of media and methods in occupational therapy. Eight factors are identified: cultural, social, economic, political, technological, theoretical, historical, and research. The effects of these eight factors are summarized in 14 assumptions. Three examples—arts and crafts, sanding blocks, and work-related programs—are used to illustrate the factors and assumptions. It is recommended that an improved approach to occupational analysis be used based on values and interests to understand why occupational therapists select or discard specific media and methods.

33. Allen, C. K. (1987). Activity: Occupational therapy's treatment method. *Am J Occup Ther, 41,* 563-75.

Keywords: activity, environment

This Eleanor Clarke Slagle lecture focuses on activity, particularly as it is related to the definition of disability, which is the inability to do a certain activity. She describes activity as a medium through which humans interact with the environment (human and nonhuman), and as "bits of life" used to overcome problems associated with disability. An occupational therapist's role is to analyze an activity with accuracy and precision and identify where adjustments, necessitated by the limitations of a disability, can be made.

34. Evans, K. (1987). Definition of occupation as the core concept of occupational therapy. *Am J Occup Ther, 41,* 627-628.

Keywords: essence, monism

The purpose of this brief paper is to clarify the use of the term *occupation.* The American Occupational Therapy Association's definition of occupation is "the active or doing process of a person engaged in goal-directed, intrinsically gratifying and culturally appropriate activity." The author reviews some of the basic propositions about the meaning of occupation to clarify the concept. These underlying concepts include hierarchy and developmental sequence of occupation, biopsychosocial unity, and the adaptive capacities of the human organism.

35. Levine, R. (1987). The influence of the arts-and-crafts movement on the professional status of occupational therapy. *Am J Occup Ther, 41,* 248-254.

Keywords: activity, values

This article explores the reasons occupational therapists use arts and crafts as therapeutic modalities. The author concludes that the founders of occupational therapy were responding to emerging health care issues, while the arts-and-crafts proponents continued to focus on their original ideals. The occupational therapy profession has paid a price for using arts and crafts as a therapeutic modality, as it was part of a lay health movement and resulted in conflict and confusion within the profession.

---

36. McClain, L. (1987). The challenge: Substantiating knowledge claims. *Am J Occup Ther, 41*(9), 607-609.

Keywords: knowledge, science

The author proposes that the primary concern of occupational therapy in the 1980s should be epistemology. The article suggests that the profession's values and reality are solidly founded, but it is in a crisis due to a lack of agreement of a knowledge base. New strategies to deal with new health care issues are suggested: adopting more analytic approaches to service delivery, research focusing on enhancing the knowledge base of occupational therapy, and a pragmatic approach to the development of the science of occupational therapy.

---

37. Miller, L., & Nelson, D. L. (1987). Dual purpose activity versus single-purpose activity in terms of duration of task, exertion level and affect. *Occupational Therapy in Mental Health, 7*, 55-67.

Keyword: activity

The article begins with a thorough discussion of the notion of purposeful activity, its features, and effects. A study is then reported that examines purposeful activity versus exercise in a sample of college undergraduates. The study shows that subjects evaluate purposeful activity more favourably, although they may not particularly exert themselves more.

---

38. Friedland, J. (1988). Diversional activity: Does it deserve its bad name? *Am J Occup Ther, 42*, 603-608.

Keywords: activity, history

This article reviews the concept of diversional activity, as originally found in occupational therapy literature, and relates it to current treatment rationales. Diversionary activity is a commonplace tool for treatment that has existed for centuries and was recognized as important by our founders. The concept of diversional activity deserves to be researched more thoroughly as the profession of occupational therapy reaffirms the concept of occupation. The author concludes that diversional activity should maintain a small but important place in the practice of occupational therapy.

---

39. Henderson, A. (1988). Occupational therapy knowledge: From practice to theory. *Am J Occup Ther, 42*, 567-576.

Keywords: knowledge, technology

This article asserts that technology in occupational therapy is an important source for theory. Occupational therapy technology is defined as "our body of knowledge of assessment and intervention techniques." The author discusses three topics related to technology: (1) knowledge of technology should be given equal value to philosophical knowledge, (2) the development of technology can take place in practice through theory development and research, and (3) the development of technology is evident throughout the history of occupational therapy, particularly as it relates to the manipulation of objects.

40. Nelson, D. (1988). Occupation: Form and performance. *Am J Occup Ther, 42,* 633-641.

Keywords: models, terminology

The author attempts to eliminate ambiguity in the term *occupation* by defining two additional terms: occupational form, referring to the pre-existing structure or circumstances that are external to a person, and occupational performance, referring to objectively observable human actions taken in the context of an occupational form. The relationships between occupational form and occupational performance are dynamic, not deterministic.

41. Yerxa, E. J. (1988). Oversimplification: The hobgoblin of theory and practice in occupational therapy. *Canadian Journal of Occupational Therapy, 55,* 5-6.

Keywords: pluralism, systems

The author suggests that occupational therapy, in response to medical and societal reductionism, is at risk of oversimplification, where complex phenomena are reduced to parts or fragments. She reminds us that the essential quality of occupational therapy is the complexity of knowledge and practice. Occupational therapy must deal with many levels of function of the human system to be truly occupational. Some of these hierarchical levels are described briefly to support the argument that occupation is too important to be oversimplified.

42. McCuaig, M., & Iwama, M. (1989). When daily living becomes a challenge in the workplace. Occupational therapy: The profession that connects. *Canadian Journal of Occupational Therapy, 56,* 161-162.

Keywords: environment, work

The authors address the challenge occupational therapists are facing in addressing the complex connection between a worker's skills and employment opportunities. They focus on the philosophy of the profession regarding productivity and discuss present and future roles for occupational therapists.

43. Christiansen, C. (1990). The perils of plurality. *Occupational Therapy Journal of Research, 10,* 259-265.

Keywords: knowledge, monism

In this editorial, the author examines and attempts to refute many of the reasons used by occupational therapists to justify pluralism. It is argued that a pluralistic approach actively fosters diversity at the expense of progress in developing occupational therapy as an applied science. A unified structure is suggested to enhance our understanding of the role of occupation in the health and well-being of humankind.

44. Yerxa, E., Clark, F., Frank, G., Jackson, J., Parham, D., Pierce, D., et al. (1990). An introduction to occupational science, a foundation for occupational therapy in the 21st century. *Occupational Therapy in Health Care, 6(4),* 1-17.

Keywords: history, science

Yerxa and colleagues discuss occupational science as "an emerging basic science," with occupation as its central construct. They define and discuss occupation and its relationship to health from both a historical and a contemporary standpoint. Finally, they outline an agenda for research on occupation as a basic science.

45. Clark, F. (1991). Occupational science: Academic innovation in the service of occupational therapy's future. *Am J Occup Ther, 45,* 300-310.

Keywords: education, science

Occupational science is defined as the systematic study of humans as occupational beings. Concepts and principles of occupational science are discussed, with particular reference to other social and health science. The article also advances a proposal for doctoral-level education of occupational scientists.

46. Schkade, J. K., & Schultz, S. (1992). Occupational adaptation: Toward a holistic approach for contemporary practice. Part 1. *Am J Occup Ther, 46,* 829-837.

Keywords: adaptation, environment

This is the first of two articles advancing a frame of reference for occupational therapy. It begins with the assumptions that occupation is the vehicle for adaptation. Occupational adaptation is therefore a process that is nonhierarchical and non-stage-specific, whereby internal and external experiences contribute to functional changes aimed at mastery.

47. Kielhofner, G. (1992). *Conceptual foundations of occupational therapy.* Philadelphia: F. A. Davis.

Keyword: models

In this book, Kielhofner advances a model similar to the one used in this book to organize the body of knowledge guiding occupational therapy. The central paradigm, which consists of the profession's basic values, is surrounded by conceptual practice models and related knowledge from other disciplines.

48. Mosey, A. C. (1992). Partition of occupational science and occupational therapy. *Am J Occup Ther, 46,* 851-853.

Keywords: knowledge, science

Mosey begins by noting that the development of scientific discipline out of a practice profession is unprecedented in the scientific community. She advocates for the partition, meaning a complete split between the discipline of occupational science and the profession of occupational therapy, as a means of ensuring the optimum success of each.

49. Polatajko, H. J. (1992). Naming and framing occupational therapy: A lecture dedicated to the life of Nancy B. *Canadian Journal of Occupational Therapy, 59,* 189-198.

Keywords: competence, disability

In this Muriel Driver Memorial Lecture, Polatajko ties together the concepts of occupation and disability by proposing a model of enablement. Enablement is defined as occupational competence used to overcome disability and handicap. Occupational competence is achieved through the interaction of ability and environment.

50. Clark, F. (1993). Occupation embedded in a real life: Interweaving occupational science and occupational therapy. *Am J Occup Ther, 47,* 1067-1078.

Keywords: phenomenology, science

This paper presents occupation as phenomenology, as experience. It recommends a number of qualitative research approaches for this aspect of occupational science. In particular, the article emphasizes story telling and narrative as a means of understanding the phenomenological aspect of occupation.

51. Llorens, L. (1993). Activity analysis: Agreement between participants and observers on perceived factors in occupational components. *Occupational Therapy Journal of Research, 13,* 198-211.

Keywords: activity, phenomenology

The article presents a study looking at the percent agreement between participants and observers in five occupations. Each occupation was rated according to 29 factors, and a moderate amount of concordance was achieved between observers and participants. This finding is interpreted in terms of the experience of occupation, which cannot be observed.

---

52. Miller, R. J., & Walker, K. F. (1993). *Perspectives on theory for the practice of occupational therapy.* Gaithersberg, MD: Aspen.

Keyword: knowledge

This book expands on a previous volume by the same authors, entitled *Six Perspectives on Theory.* It reviews the work and contributions of seven prominent American occupational therapy theorists: Claudia Allen, Jean Ayres, Gail Fidler, Gary Kielhofner, Lela Llorens, Anne Mosey, and Mary Reilly.

---

53. Wood, W. (1993). Occupation and the relevance of primatology to occupational therapy. *Am J Occup Ther, 47,* 515-522.

Keywords: essence, science

This paper presents a review of research about occupation and its capacity to promote occupation in nonhuman primates and the links to our understanding of the nature of occupation in humans. Phylogenetic and ontogenetic perspectives demonstrate the need for occupational engagement in the development of the species as well as the individual. The author concludes that occupation is a feature of primates and is therefore "hard-wired" in human ontogeny. This review is used to suggest an agenda for research in occupational science.

---

54. Yerxa, E. (1993). Occupational science: A new source of power for participants in occupational therapy. *Journal of Occupational Science (Australia), 1,* 3-10.

Keywords: education, science

The definition and tenets of occupational science are discussed, with particular reference to the assumptions that underlie it. Occupational science is discussed in terms of its potential for consolidating the power and legitimacy of occupational therapy in health care, education, and policy.

---

55. Christiansen, C. (1994). Classification and study in occupation: A review and discussion of taxonomies. *Journal of Occupational Science (Australia), 1,* 3-21.

Keywords: models, science

The paper advances the need for a classification system for occupational science knowledge if its development is to proceed successfully. Several taxonomies from other disciplines are considered in recognition of the broad reach of theory underlying the study of occupation.

56. Trombly, C. A. (1995). Occupation: Purposefulness and meaning-fulness as therapeutic mechanisms. *Am J Occup Ther, 49,* 44-52.

Keywords: activity, phenomenology

This lecture defines two important ideas in occupational therapy: purposefulness, referring to the outcome of an activity, and meaningfulness, referring to the motivational quality of an activity. These two qualities are identified with occupations that are viewed as the goal of therapy (*ends*) and occupations that are used in the process of therapy (*means*).

57. Wood, W. (1995). The warp and weft of occupational therapy: An art & science for all times. *Am J Occup Ther, 49,* 44-52.

Keywords: activity, humanism, values

The article uses the metaphor of weaving to explore the art and science of occupational therapy. The warp is the basic belief that engagement in occupation is health promoting; the weft is equated with the humanistic value of the person. These two weave together to produce a tapestry of human potential.

58. Law, M., Cooper, B., Strong, S., Stewart, D., Rigby, P., & Letts, L. (1996). The person-environment-occupation model: A transactive approach to occupational performance. *Canadian Journal of Occupational Therapy, 63,* 9-23.

Keywords: environment, models

This model focuses on the transactional nature of the relationship between person, occupation, and environment. It defines occupational performance as this dynamic interaction and occupation as clusters of activities and tasks involved in carrying out a role.

59. Zemke, R., & Clark, F. (1996). *Occupational science: The evolving discipline.* Philadelphia: F. A. Davis.

Keywords: knowledge, science

This book is a collection of essays representing the development of the discipline of occupational therapy. Most impressive about this volume is its breadth of scope and the range of disciplines from which its contributors are drawn. They include such renowned scientists as Jane Goodall and Stephen Hawking.

60. Canadian Association of Occupational Therapists (1997). *Enabling occupation.* Ottawa, ON: CAOT ACE.

Keyword: models

This is the third edition of Canada's national guidelines for the practice of occupational therapy, with substantial revisions to the basic model and concepts.

Occupational performance is defined as the ability to choose, organize, and satisfactorily perform meaningful occupations that are culturally defined and age appropriate. Occupations include looking after oneself, enjoying life, and contributing to the social and economic fabric of the community.

61. Christiansen, C., & Baum, C. (Eds.). (1997). *Occupational therapy: Enabling function and well-being* (2nd ed.). Thorofare, NJ: SLACK Incorporated.

Keywords: hierarchy, models

In this second edition of their book, Christiansen and Baum advance a model of occupational performance made up of intrinsic (biological and psychological) factors and extrinsic (social and cultural) factors. They equate occupational performance with function in a hierarchical model of identity, roles, tasks, and actions.

62. Clark, F. (1997). Reflections on the human as an occupational being: Biological need, tempo, and temporality. *Journal of Occupational Science (Australia), 4, 86-92.*

Keywords: essence, history, time

This paper is based on two fundamental assumptions: that humans have a biological need for occupation, and that occupation is profoundly influenced by time. Clark traces the occupation of prehistoric humans to learn lessons about its health-promoting potential.

63. Emerson, H. (1998). Flow and occupation: A review of the literature. *Canadian Journal of Occupational Therapy, 65, 37-44.*

Keywords: activity, phenomenology

This paper uses the concept of flow, advanced by Csikszentmihalyi, to describe the state of being totally involved in an activity or occupation. The characteristics of this state are elaborated, and the literature is reviewed for evidence of flow experiences in therapy. The paper concludes by suggesting a research agenda.

64. Kielhofner, G., & Barrett, L. (1998). Meaning and misunderstanding in occupational forms: A study of therapeutic goal-setting. *Am J Occup Ther, 52, 345-353.*

Keywords: phenomenology, therapeutic relationship

This article reports the results of a qualitative study of the relationship between therapist and client narratives of therapy. The authors found that therapists created a narrative of the occupational form or the context for occupational performance that they hoped to establish in therapy. At the same time, clients created a personal volitional narrative grounded in their own socio-cultural context. When these two narratives did not coincide, the therapeutic relationship was characterized by difficulties.

65. Law, M. (1998). *Client-centered occupational therapy.* Thorofare, NJ: SLACK Incorporated.

Keywords: therapeutic relationship

This edited volume is a basic textbook on client-centred practice in occupational therapy, from concept to implementation.

66. Law, M., Steinwender, S., & LeClair, L. (1998). Occupation, health and well-being. *Canadian Journal of Occupational Therapy, 65,* 81-91.

Keywords: essence, science

This article offers a quantitative analysis of the literature of occupation and health to estimate the strength of the relationship between occupation and health. Using 22 studies involving people with disabilities, published in the last decade, the authors conclude that there is "moderate to strong evidence" for the effect of occupation on health and well-being.

67. McLaughlin Gray, J. (1998). Putting occupation into practice: Occupation as ends, occupation as means. *Am J Occup Ther, 52,* 354-364.

Keyword: activity

The article is a response to the perceived difficulty that occupational therapists have in maintaining occupation (rather than performance components) as the focus of therapy. The author makes use of Trombly's idea of occupation as both means and ends, and interprets these ideas for use in practice.

68. Neistadt, M. E., & Crepeau, E. B. (1998). *Willard & Spackman's occupational therapy* (9th ed.). Philadelphia: Lippincott.

Keywords: knowledge, science

This is the ninth edition of a classic occupational therapy textbook, which was first published in 1954. It begins with an introduction to occupational therapy and occupational science, and proceeds to focus on elements of the occupational therapy process. It defines occupational science in terms of form, function, and meaning in occupation.

69. Pierce, D. (1998). What is the source of occupation's treatment power. *Am J Occup Ther, 52,* 490-491.

Keywords: activity, values

This brief article assumes the power of occupation as a therapeutic medium, and explores the origins of that power. Pierce advances three characteristics that she credits with the power to effect changes in treatment: occupational appeal, meaning the desirability or attractiveness of an occupation; occupational intactness, meaning the consistency of the therapeutic occupation with its naturally occurring counterpart; and goal fit, meaning the extent to which a therapeutic occupation is compatible with the patient's goal.

---

70. **Wilcock, A. A. (1998). Reflections on doing, being, and becoming.** *Canadian Journal of Occupational Therapy, 65, 240-256.*

Keywords: essence, identity

In this article, occupation is defined as a synthesis of doing, being, and becoming. Wilcock underlines the essential nature of doing for occupational therapy and defines being as the establishment of identity and authenticity. These two concepts are linked with the process of becoming. Wilcock illustrates the synthesis of these three with several anecdotal examples.

---

71. **Wilcock, A. A. (1998).** *An occupational perspective on health.* **Thorofare, NJ: SLACK Incorporated.**

Keyword: essence

This book conceptualizes occupation as part of a three-part equation for survival. It views health, occupation, and survival as inextricably linked. Health is viewed as the successful meeting of sustenance and safety needs, and occupation is the vehicle through which these needs are met.

---

72. **Yerxa, E. J. (1998). Occupation: The keystone of a curriculum for a self-defined profession.** *Am J Occup Ther, 52, 365-372.*

Keywords: education, knowledge, monism

Yerxa contemplates the implications of educating occupational therapists in an occupation-centred curriculum, as part of a curriculum renaissance for the new millennium.

---

73. **Yerxa, E. J. (1998). Health and the human spirit for occupation.** *Am J Occup Ther, 52, 412-418.*

Keywords: education, essence

The article explores the relationship between occupation and health, including the health of those with chronic impairments. Yerxa posits a relationship between occupation and survival, based on reviews of the literature. She entreats occupational therapists to become more ardent students of humans and their occupations.

74. American Occupational Therapy Association. (1999). Scope of occupational therapy. *Am J Occup Ther, 53*, 258-262.

Keyword: activity

In a special publication by the AOTA defining the scope and process of occupational therapy, occupations are defined as "goal-directed pursuits which typically extend over time, have meaning to the performer, and involve multiple tasks…[they are] the ordinary and familiar things that people do every day."

75. Christiansen, C. (1999). Defining lives: Occupation as identity. An essay on competence, coherence, and the creation of meaning. *Am J Occup Ther, 53*, 547-558.

Keywords: identity, time

This Eleanor Clark Slagle lecture advances the idea that identity is the mechanism through which occupation affects health. Identity is understood in terms of its relationship to the past, the present, and the future for an individual, and occupational therapy practitioners are encouraged to assist clients address identity as a means to overcome disability and promote health.

76. Christiansen, C., Little, B., & Backman, C. (1999). Personal projects: A useful approach to the study of occupation. *Am J Occup Ther, 53*, 439-446.

Keywords: activity, identity

Christiansen and colleagues offer a new way of understanding occupations, as a means for expression of the self, and through formation and maintenance of identity. They define personal projects as examples of complex occupations, meaning activities aimed at a personal goal, such as learning to play the piano, overcoming one's fear of meeting new people, and finding out about one's ancestors.

77. Reed, K. L., & Sanderson, S. N. (1999). *Concepts of occupational therapy* (4th ed.). Philadelphia: Lippincott Williams & Wilkins.

Keywords: knowledge, models, philosophy

This is the fourth edition of this overview of theory and ideology in occupational therapy. It divides the epistemology of occupational therapy into philosophy, concepts, consumer domain, models, knowledge, skills, practice, and history.

78. Ribeiro, K. L., & Polgar, J. M. (1999). Enabling occupational performance: Optimal experiences in therapy. *Canadian Journal of Occupational Therapy, 66*, 14-22.

Keywords: environment, phenomenology

This article reviews the concept of optimal experience and suggests that it is comparable to the experience of flow that may be experienced in conjunction with occupation. The authors suggest that the "just-right challenge" from the environment is essential for optimal experience. They encourage occupational therapists to explore these aspects for application to therapy.

79. Sumsion, T. (1999). *Client-centred practice in occupational therapy: A guide to implementation.* Edinburgh, Scotland: Churchill Livingstone.

Keywords: therapeutic relationship

This is an edited volume examining issues in various arenas of practice for the implementation of a client-centred approach to occupational therapy practice.

80. Fearing, V. G., & Clark, J. (2000). *Individuals in context: A practical guide to client-centered practice.* Thorofare, NJ: SLACK Incorporated.

Keywords: environment, therapeutic relationship

This is a third edited volume for practitioners that elaborates a model of the process of occupational therapy based on concepts of client-centred practice, leadership, and the environment/context.

81. Punwar, A., & Peloquin, S. M. (2000). *Occupational therapy: Principles and practice* (3rd ed.). Philadelphia: Lippincott Williams & Wilkins.

Keyword: knowledge

This is the third edition of a book that focuses on the practice of occupational therapy in various speciality areas and practice arenas.

82. Whiteford, G. (2000). Occupational deprivation: Global challenge in the new millennium. *British Journal of Occupational Therapy, 64,* 200-210.

Keywords: environment, values

This article takes an international perspective on a concept that the author defines and clarifies, specifically occupational deprivation. Occupational deprivation is the experience of being prevented from participating in occupation by external forces. Whiteford predicts that social, economic, and political forces will increase the incidence of occupational deprivation, making an occupational justice perspective more important for occupational therapists.

8 HOW OCCUPATION CHANGES

Nancy Pollock, MSc and Mary Ann McColl, PhD

In the first chapter, we stated that there were three principles upon which the literature in occupational therapy seems unanimous: that occupation is essential to humans, that it changes to meet internal and external demands, and that it can be used therapeutically to promote health. In this chapter, we focus on the second of those three tenets and look at what occupational therapists know about how occupation changes.

Occupational therapists are inextricably involved in the process of change. By definition, therapy involves change. Yet many therapists are neither clear nor comfortable with the notion of change or with their role as an agent of change. They worry that to participate in change means to impose one's will on another, to exercise power over another, or to undermine the autonomy of another. While these are all worthy and valid considerations, change is an integral component of therapy. People do not seek the support and assistance of a therapist unless they intend (whether implicitly or explicitly) to make a change. Therefore, it is essential for occupational therapists to understand the process of change and to have theoretical tools for thinking about change.

There are three basic processes found in the literature to describe how occupation changes: development, adaptation, and accommodation. Development refers to an intrinsically programmed change in occupation that is sequential and predictable; adaptation refers to a behavioural change aimed at achieving mastery within the environment; and accommodation refers to changes in the environment to support occupation. There has been both conflict and confusion among these ideas (primarily the first two) over the decades, and we will attempt in this chapter to clarify these concepts and reconcile ideas associated with each.

Development

First, let us clarify some of the terminology that may have led to this confusion. The word *development* has been used in occupational therapy literature to refer to changes in occupation that happen over time, or that involve a lifespan perspective. In this chapter, we will expand the lifespan perspective to allow us to differentiate development from two other concepts: maturation and adaptation. We define maturation as a biologically determined process of change that happens to the organism even in the absence of outside influences (Mosey, 1986). For hypothetical purposes only, we imagine a process whereby if a baby was isolated from all external influences, he or she would still change in some unavoidable ways—he or she would not remain a newborn perpetually. This process we call maturation, and we acknowledge that it is intrinsic, passive, sequential, and predictable. The organism is hardwired to undergo these changes.

However what complicates things is that we do not raise babies in bell-jars, sequestered from outside influences. Instead they are constantly exposed to influences from the environment. Therefore, we need another term to talk about the effect of the environment, and another for the cumulative effect of biology and environment. We will use the terms *adaptation* and *development* to refer to these two processes respectively. Furthermore, we acknowledge that we sometimes want to talk about how people change over the lifespan without necessarily invoking one of these processes. For those situations, we will attempt to talk about lifespan processes in general.

Perhaps the most controversial of the processes discussed in this chapter is development. At the beginning of the period covered in this book, there were numerous schemes and schedules describing how different components of the individual developed. Throughout the 1900s, detailed lists emerged to characterize the physical, social, cognitive, psychosexual, and moral development of the human organism. It was assumed that development was natural, pre-programmed, fixed, and hierarchical. Further, it was assumed that recovery must replicate development if it was to have any hope of success.

More recent literature has called into question some of these assumptions. Work done primarily in the area of motor development has suggested that the typical sequence of changes seen in human motor development may not be as pre-programmed as previously believed. It is suggested that these changes may be a response by the organism to changes in physical characteristics (e.g., weight, limb length) coupled with the innate drive to find the optimal movement solution. The emergence of dynamic system models has moved our thinking about development away from hierarchical models toward models that account for the influence of the interaction of multiple systems on behaviour, including body systems, environmental demands, and the nature of the task. Thus, it came to be understood that development occurred not only longitudinally, or vertically, over time. It also occurred horizontally, meaning across systems of the human being. It was a complex interaction of many factors both within and outside the individual.

These newer theories of development raise serious questions about some models of practice, particularly those that became most prevalent in neurological rehabilitation based on a hierarchical view of development. These theories also shift the balance between nature and nurture or between maturation and adaptation. They place more weight on skill acquisition as a function of the drive to adapt, with maturation being only one of the ingredients to be considered in the interaction between humans and environments.

There may also be some value in thinking about the predominance of the maturation factor at different stages throughout the lifespan. Biological maturation is very rapid during the first few years of life and often comes to the fore again late in life, when functional losses may occur as a result of aging. During the extended middle period of the lifespan, adaptation is most likely the main route through which occupation changes. While maturational change is arguably still present among adults, it is likely to be very subtle.

Adaptation

In the early 1960s, the concept of adaptation gained popularity in psychological literature, and it was but a short step from there to the occupational therapy literature. White's 1971 *American Journal of Occupational Therapy* article, entitled "The Urge Towards Competence," introduced the idea that humans are motivated to master their environments. Thus, the idea of purposeful adaptation emerged, in which individuals make strategic strides toward behaviours that support their functioning and problem solving in response to particular environmental challenges. This extrinsic approach to development flew in the face of contemporary ideas about development, which emphasized the intrinsic pre-programmed development of the human organism.

Unlike maturation, which is motivated intrinsically and initiated subconsciously, adaptation is defined as purposeful and intentional. It is an active strategy aimed at achieving mastery, which becomes integrated subcortically only after it has been shown to be successful. Adaptation is most prevalent in adolescent and adult development, when the opportunity for purposeful action is greatest. Adaptive responses are self-reinforcing in that they produce the desired outcome, which is mastery. In addition, adaptive responses change the human organism itself, increasing its capacity to respond effectively to future challenges.

Adaptation can occur at three levels. Some authors talk about evolutionary adaptation, meaning adaptive changes that occur throughout the existence of the species; others deal with ontogenetic adaptation, meaning changes occurring over the lifetime of the individual; and finally, others refer to immediate or situational adaptation in response to a particular problem. To further complicate the picture, the word adaptation takes on different forms of speech in occupational therapy. It is used as a verb, denoting a process; as an abstract noun, denoting an outcome; and as a concrete noun, denoting a modification, such as an aid or assistive device. Adaptation is a word that is pervasive in definitions and descriptions of occupational therapy, and yet there is some confusion about exactly what it is.

Accommodation

The concept of accommodation is found in the occupational therapy literature in the 1990s, as the socio-political definition of disability gained prevalence. This definition of disability emphasizes the idea that disability is socially constructed, defined, and perpetuated by society and social institutions. It focuses on the role of the environment in the determination of disability. Accommodation refers to changes made to the environment in order to provide equal opportunities to people with disabilities. Accommodations are often undertaken to meet the requirements of a specific individual, however they represent changes to the environment rather than the person.

Accommodations are differentiated from adaptive devices in that adaptive devices are proximal to the individual and travel with him or her to different environments. Accommodations tend to be more distal to the individual and are specific to a particular environment. Thus while a customized typing device may be considered an adaptive device because it is applied by the individual and travels with him or her to various different keyboards, an adapted workstation would be considered an accommodation, because it is a change to the environment that is distal to the individual and specific to the particular office environment.

Table 8-1 — Theoretical Tools Associated With Change in Occupation

	DEVELOPMENT	ADAPTATION	ACCOMMODATION
OCCUPATIONAL CONCEPTUAL MODELS	Ways of understanding change in occupation as a function of intrinsically programmed change in the person (e.g., Mosey's *Recapitulation of Ontogenesis*)	Ways of understanding change in occupation as a function of interaction with the environment (e.g., Schkade & Schultz's occupational adaptation)	Ways of understanding how occupation changes when the environment changes (e.g., person-environment-occupation model)
BASIC CONCEPTUAL MODELS	Ways of understanding how the component areas of the human organism develop (e.g., Freud, Erikson, Kohlberg)	Ways of understanding how human beings change in response to the environment (e.g., dynamic systems theory)	Ways of understanding how other aspects of human beings change in response to changes in the environment (e.g., independent living)
OCCUPATIONAL MODELS OF PRACTICE	Ways of promoting change in occupation that are consistent with intrinsically programmed change (e.g., Llorens, Gilfoyle & Grady)	Ways of promoting change in occupation through interactions with the environment (e.g., activity analysis, occupational adaptation)	Ways of promoting change in occupation by making changes in the environment (e.g., universal design)
BASIC MODELS OF PRACTICE	Ways of affecting how the the components of human beings develop (e.g., sensory integration, Piaget)	Ways of affecting other types of human functioning through interactions with the environment (e.g., environmental press, the just-right challenge)	Ways of affecting human performance components by altering the environment (e.g., urban planning)

According to this perspective, occupation among people with disabilities changes when the environment changes to permit or support it. The Americans with Disabilities Act of 1990 in the United States provided a further stimulus for American occupational therapists to think about how occupation changes when accommodations are put in place. The act became a legislative imperative for all of American society, including occupational therapy, to give greater consideration to altering occupation by putting in place reasonable accommodations.

Table 8-1 summarizes the theory associated with each of these modes of change in occupation, with examples of theoretical ideas associated with each. It shows how change is conceptualized in occupational conceptual models, occupational models of practice, basic conceptual models, and basic models of practice. In other words, it looks at how the toolbox is equipped to deal with change in occupation.

KEYWORDS USED IN THIS CHAPTER			
Accommodation	Competence	Knowledge	Systems
Adaptation	Coping	Lifespan	Terminology
Adolescents	Development	Models	Time
Adults	Disability	Philosophy	Values
Aging	Environment	Physical	Work
Biopsychosocial	Hierarchy	Play	
Children	History	Process	
Cognition	Identity	Science	

Bibliographic References
Associated With Three Types of Change

Following are references associated with each of the three types of change in occupation, and classified according to the keywords below.

DEVELOPMENT

83. Fiorentino, M. (1975). Occupational therapy: Realization to activation. *Am J Occup Ther, 29*, 15-21.

Keywords: children, development

This article presents the author's views of the growth and development of paediatric occupational therapy as it relates to the habilitation and rehabilitation of children with physical disabilities. A parallel is drawn between a child's development and an adult's professional development. An overview of the process of occupational therapy demonstrates that we need to move from "realization to activation" so that the role of occupational therapy can be accepted as a vital part of the rehabilitation of the child.

84. Black, M. (1976). Adolescent role assessment. *Am J Occup Ther, 30*, 73-80.

Keywords: adolescents, development

Adolescence is a complex period when children are expected to shed their dependencies and achieve a level of independence as adults. Frequently, adult independence is achieved through the occupational role where individuals recognize personal assets and liabilities and participate cooperatively in society. The decision-making process that guides adolescents in the search for an occupational role is occupational choice. This paper traces the development of skills necessary for the occupational choice process.

85. **Woodside, H. (1976). Dimensions of the occupational behaviour model.** *Canadian Journal of Occupational Therapy, 43, 11-14.*

Keywords: development, play, work

The article gives a theoretical outline of the occupational behaviour model that is used in an in-patient psychiatric service. Occupational behaviour is described as the developmental continuum of play and work. The effects of developmental gaps and institutionalization on a person's occupational behaviour are explored. It is concluded that the occupational behaviour model can be used by occupational therapists to help their clients support and build the skills "necessary and inherent" in each individual.

86. **Llorens, L. (1977). A developmental theory revisited.** *Am J Occup Ther, 31, 656-657.*

Keywords: development, history, knowledge

In this brief article, the author takes a retrospective look at the Eleanor Clarke Slagle lecture she presented in 1969. A theoretical framework of facilitating growth and development is expanded on, and the work conducted by the author since 1969 is outlined. An emerging teaching technique called *developmental analysis* is defined as the analytical step in the therapy process in which occupational therapists mentally scan their knowledge and theory base to recognize possible problem areas prior to client evaluation.

87. **Robinson, A. L. (1977). Play: the arena for acquisition of rules for competent behavior.** *Am J Occup Ther, 31, 248-253.*

Keywords: children, development, play

The article identifies play as the critical arena for learning rules. A rule is defined as a symbol, which governs action by defining the plan for execution. Preliminary questions about the clinical application of play and rules are explored. It is suggested that occupational therapists can organize their observations of play based on the information gained from this study. The complexity of the phenomenon of play is recognized as is the process of nurturing play. Play is viewed as a complex process in which individuals process information from the environment.

88. **Woodside, H. (1977). A developmental perspective.** *Canadian Journal of Occupational Therapy, 44, 131-135.*

Keywords: development, models, play

A brief outline of what is meant by a developmental perspective is considered prior to examining its application to occupational therapy. Development concepts useful to practitioners are considered. This is followed by a review of the two present theories developed by occupational therapists that are based on developmental models. This information is given as a basis for the main objective of the paper: to propose a developmental perspective for occupational therapy based on play behaviour. A continuum of play behaviour is traced through four general phases of life to illustrate this model.

---

89. **Clark, P. N. (1979). Human development through occupation: Theoretical frameworks in contemporary occupational therapy practice. Part 1.** *Am J Occup Ther, 33,* 505-514.

Keywords: development, knowledge, models

This article presents four significant theoretical frameworks for occupational therapy. The concepts of Fidler and Mosey are combined together as *adaptive performance.* Llorens' concepts of *facilitating growth and development* and the work of several theorists that studied the *biodevelopmental* or neuromotor components of performance are discussed. Finally, Reilly's work on *occupational behaviour* is presented. A model for the analysis of theory is also outlined and the four theoretical frameworks are summarized using this model.

---

90. **Clark, P. N. (1979). Human development through occupation: A philosophy and conceptual model for practice. Part 2.** *Am J Occup Ther, 33,* 577-585.

Keywords: activity, development, philosophy

This article describes a philosophy of occupational therapy practice that is named *human development through occupation.* It is a philosophy that unites, and is derived from, the generic concepts of four theoretical frameworks that dominate current occupational therapy practice. The philosophy is described in terms of a view of man, a view of health, and a view of the profession. A conceptual model of the process of occupational therapy is then proposed based on this philosophy. Examples of application are included and suggestions for further research are given.

---

91. **Gratz, R. R., & Zemke, R. (1980). Piaget, preschoolers, and paediatric practice.** *Physical and Occupational Therapy in Paediatrics, 1,* 3-9.

Keywords: cognition, development, children

The authors attempt to apply Piaget's cognitive approach to occupational therapy. Several of the major characteristics of Piaget's theory that are unique to the preschool child are described. They include egocentrism, centration, irreversibility and reasoning. Suggestions are then given about how these concepts may be applied in a paediatric setting. It is concluded that application of Piagetian theory can be an excellent aid to therapy.

92. Kielhofner, G. (1980). A model of human occupation. Part 2. Ontogenesis from the perspective of temporal adaptation. *Am J Occup Ther, 34, 657-663.*

Keywords: development, systems, time

This article is the second in a series that presents a model of human occupation. It adds to the model a description of how occupation evolves throughout the lifespan and an explanation of the process of change. The systems concept of hierarchy is used as a foundation for explaining the process of ontogenesis or change. Occupational behaviour over the lifespan of an individual is discussed according to the perspective of temporal adaptation. The characterization of work and play over the four life stages is presented as a major element in this process.

93. Menks, F. (1980). Changes and challenges of mid life. Part 1. A review of the literature. *Occupational Therapy in Mental Health, 1, 15-28.*

Keywords: adult, development, identity

This article reviews the developmental literature on middle adulthood and describes some of the main physical and psychosocial changes that occur. Critical psychological issues are identified that evolve from the re-evaluation of former goals, values, and achievements. These issues are related to the time-left orientation characteristic of mid life. Socio-cultural changes involving new developmental stages in the family, work, and leisure are discussed. Changes in physical and cognitive capacities and functions are described. These changes are regarded as crisis since they challenge the individual with options that can lead to further individuation and life satisfaction.

94. Florey, L. (1981). Studies of play: Implications for growth, development, and for clinical practice. *Am J Occup Ther, 35, 519-524.*

Keywords: children, development, play

This article summarizes some of the studies of play conducted by graduate students in occupational therapy. The overall boundaries and clinical yields of these studies of play are identified. The author acknowledges the theme of growth and development in play as a common theme in all studies. The concepts of open systems and hierarchy are used to help understand the process of change in growth and development in play. Three main clinical tasks for occupational therapists are identified: observation of a child's play, a history of the child's play, and setting up a milieu for intervention in play.

95. Vandenberg, B., & Kielhofner, G. (1982). Play in evolution, cultural and individual adaptation: Implications for therapy. *Am J Occup Ther, 36, 20-28.*

Keywords: development, hierarchy, play

The purpose of this article is to present a theoretical basis for occupational therapists to understand the role of play in human development and functioning. The author describes evolutionary, cultural, and ontogenetic perspectives of play in order to demonstrate how it affects human beings throughout their lifespan. It is proposed that play might be conceptualized as a critical element in the adaptation process of the patient and as a tool for therapy. Examples of the potential of play in the areas of physical disabilities and psychosocial dysfunction are given.

96. Zemke, R. (1982). The role of theory: Erikson and occupational therapy. *Occupational Therapy in Mental Health, 2, 45-64.*

Keywords: development, knowledge, models

In his psychosocial theory of development, Erik Erikson poses a viable framework from which occupational therapists may evaluate and assess adjustment to dysfunction. Occupational therapists are familiar with the application of Erikson's eight stages to developmental problems. The authors present suggestions for the application of this theory to a variety of psychosocial and physical dysfunctions affecting mental health. These problems may result in the need to resolve Eriksonian crises at later points rather than regarding each crisis from a purely age-oriented developmental view. Awareness of the role of theory in the clinical application of occupational therapists skills may suggest new approaches for the therapist.

97. Goodgold-Edwards, S. A. (1984). Motor learning as it relates to the development of skilled motor behavior: A review of the literature. *Physical and Occupational Therapy in Paediatrics, 4, 5-18.*

Keywords: development, physical

The purpose of this article is to review pertinent literature on motor learning as it relates to aspects of motor skill performance and development. The development course and evolutionary pattern of certain performance parameters are identified, including speed, accuracy, anticipation, kinaesthesia, and strategy. The rate and level of motor skill learning is viewed as a function of the characteristics of both the learner and the task. It is concluded that motor learning theory can be an important component in designing and implementing therapeutic regimes for children with disabilities.

98. Blakeney, A. B. (1985). Adolescent development: An application of the model of human occupation. *Occupational Therapy in Health Care, 2, 19-40.*

Keywords: adolescents, development, competence

The developmental stage of adolescence is discussed relative to the components of the model of human occupation. Emerging themes include the need for exploration and mastery, the development of values, the increasing variety of interests, the drive toward occupational choice and self-identity, and the development and internalization of roles.

99. **Kielhofner, G., & Barris, R. (1985). The development of occupational behaviour. In: G. Kielhofner (Ed.), *A model of human occupation: Theory and application* (pp. 78-81). Baltimore: Williams & Wilkins.**

Keywords: competence, development, lifespan

This chapter represents an introduction to a larger section of the book devoted to an examination of the development of occupational behaviour across the lifespan. The authors address the interweaving of maturation and adaptation, and highlight the importance of cultural influences and historical periods on occupational development. Subsequent chapters examine life stages from infancy to old age using the model of human occupation language of performance, habituation, and volitional subsystems. Specific roles, values, interests, and skills are described for each of the six life stages.

100. **Bruce, M. A., & Borg, B. (1987). *Frames of reference in psychosocial occupational therapy*. Thorofare, NJ: SLACK Incorporated.**

Keywords: activity, adult, development, models

This chapter presents an extensive overview of the contributions of major developmental theorists to the practice of occupational therapy with adults. Special emphasis is placed on occupational therapy theorists whose work is based on a developmental model including Mosey, Llorens, and Ayres. A discussion is included regarding mediating factors to be considered in applying developmental theory to adults and three areas of development; cognitive, sensory integrative, and moral reasoning are dealt with in more depth. The chapter explores the interrelationships among purposeful activity, development, adaptation, and a life course perspective. Examples of applications for these ideas in evaluation and treatment are also presented.

101. **Llorens, L. A. (1991). Performance tasks and roles throughout the life span. In: C. Christiansen & C. Baum (Eds.), *Occupational therapy: Overcoming human performance deficits* (pp. 45-68). Thorofare, NJ: SLACK Incorporated.**

Keywords: development, lifespan, models

This chapter provides a comprehensive overview of the contributions of major developmental theorists to our understanding of occupational performance, mastery, adaptation, and the assumption of various roles throughout the lifespan. Occupational therapy theorists are highlighted as well. The chapter moves the reader through eight life stages from infancy to old age and identifies key areas of occupational performance and occupational performance enablers. Tables provide a very succinct summary of the contributions of each theorist. Case studies facilitate the application of the concepts discussed.

102. **Coster, W. (1995). Development. In: C. A. Trombly (Ed.),** *Occupational therapy for physical dysfunction* **(pp. 255-264). Baltimore: Williams & Wilkins.**

Keywords: development, models

This chapter examines current treatment approaches that have either an explicit or implicit basis in developmental theory and questions the assumptions upon which they are based. Coster highlights some of the gaps in our knowledge of development, showing that the majority of our understanding is about the typical stages of human development and the interrelationships among various areas of development. Our understanding about the mechanisms of developmental change is quite limited and hence some of the treatment approaches used in occupational therapy may be based on flawed assumptions. The latter half of the chapter reviews some of the more contemporary theories of development including dynamic systems models and ecological psychology and considers the implications this newer understanding will have on occupational therapy interventions.

103. **Ferland, F. (1997).** *Play, children with physical disabilities and occupational therapy: The Ludic model.* **Ottawa, ON: University of Ottawa Press.**

Keywords: children, development, play

This book presents the Ludic model, a theoretical approach for occupational therapy with children, focusing on play and the therapeutic importance of play.

104. **Carlson, M., Clark, F., & Young, B. (1998). Practical contributions of occupational science to the art of successful aging: How to sculpt a meaningful life in older adulthood.** *Journal of Occupational Science, 5,* **107-118.**

Keywords: aging, development

This article, based on a lecture by Florence Clark, describes three essential ingredients for successful aging: experiencing a sense of control over one's life, practicing healthy habits, and achieving continuity with one's past. Using the results of the USC Well Elderly Research Program, the authors demonstrate the contributions that occupational therapy can make to the adoption of these health-promoting behaviours and the positive health and well-being outcomes that are possible for older persons who are well and those with illness and disability.

105. **Hinojosa, J., & Kramer, P. (1999). Developmental perspective: Fundamentals of developmental theory. In P. Kramer, & J. Hinojosa (Eds.),** *Frames of reference for pediatric occupational therapy* **(2nd ed., pp. 3-8). Baltimore: Lippincott Williams & Wilkins.**

Keywords: children, development, models

The authors propose that a thorough knowledge of human development forms the foundation upon which many of the frames of reference used in pediatric practice build. Linear models of development, where the child acquires skills in a typical progression or order, are contrasted with pyramidal or foundational models of development where skills build upon one another, with some basic skills serving as prerequisites for future skill development. The authors believe that occupational therapists use this knowledge of development to determine its impact on the child's occupational performance.

106. **Blair, S. E. E. (2000). The centrality of occupation during life transitions.** *British Journal of Occupational Therapy,* **63,** 231-237.

Keywords: adults, development, lifespan

Blair combines theory from developmental psychology with occupational science to examine occupations that are associated with adult life transitions. The author emphasizes the importance of meaning and the centrality of occupation for the successful transition between life stages.

ADAPTATION

107. **Smith, M. (1974). Competence and adaptation.** *Am J Occup Ther,* **28,** 11-15.

Keywords: adaptation, competence

Based on the work of White, published in *American Journal of Occupational Therapy* in 1970, Smith discusses the urge toward mastery as the basis for human behaviour, instead of the urge toward drive reduction. It also introduces the ideas of internal and external causation based on deCharm's ideas about pawns and origins/agents. Smith discusses benign and vicious cycles of behaviour, meaning adaptation, motivation, and competence versus helplessness, hopelessness, and maladaptation. Although this article precedes our time frame by 1 year, it is included because it introduces many important ideas that reappear throughout the period.

108. **Kielhofner, G. (1977). Temporal adaptation: A conceptual framework for occupational therapy.** *Am J Occup Ther,* **31,** 235-242.

Keywords: adaptation, time, model

The concept of temporal adaptation is reintroduced to the profession of occupational therapy, drawing on the work of Meyer and Slagle for a historical perspective on the concept. The article focuses on time as a context form of adaptive behaviour, regardless of the nature of dysfunction.

109. King, L. J. (1978). Toward a science of adaptive responses. *Am J Occup Ther, 32*, 429-437.

Keywords: adaptation, monism, science

In this Eleanor Clarke Slagle lecture, King begins with a call for a unifying theory or science of occupation. She observes that developmental frameworks, which have become so prevalent in the occupational therapy literature, are not suitable for normally developing adults and proposes a science of adaptive responses as an alternative. She discusses the concept of individual adaptation as distinct from the concept of evolutionary or species adaptation. Individual adaptation is defined as behavioural adjustments made to ensure individual survival and self-actualization. Two phases of individual adaptation are discussed: developmental learning and adaptation to stress. There are four characteristics of individual adaptation: active, elicited by the environment, organized subcortically, and self-reinforcing.

110. Kielhofner, G. (1980). A model of human occupation. Part 3. Benign and vicious cycles. *Am J Occup Ther, 34*, 731-737.

Keywords: adaptation, systems

This paper presents an explanation of adaptive and maladaptive changes in the concept of benign and vicious cycles. Hypothetical case material is used to illustrate how the model could be applied to an explanation of change in occupational behaviour. The paper also outlines how the concept of benign and vicious cycles, as conceptualized in the present model, can guide clinical intervention.

111. Gilfoyle, E. M., Grady, A. P., & Moore, J. C. (1981). *Children adapt*. Thorofare, NJ: SLACK Incorporated.

Keywords: adaptation, children

This book advances the idea that movement is central to the process of adaptation in children, and through movement, children learn about their environment and develop capabilities to deal with it. "Without movement there is not adaptation and without adaptation there is no life" (p. 1). Adaptation is defined as "a dynamic organized process of expanding a child's repertoire of behaviours" (p. 2). Adaptation occurs when automatic behaviours are purposefully adjusted to meet environmental needs and then repeated until they become automatic. Thus, it is a process of layering purposeful behaviour over automatic behaviours and using repetition to expand the repertoire of automatic behaviours.

112. Kleinman, B. L., & Buckley, B. L. (1982). Some implications of a science of adaptive responses. *Am J Occup Ther, 36*, 15-19.

Keywords: adaptation, science

These authors expand on the ideas proposed by King in 1978. They propose an adaptation continuum, consisting of homeostatic responses (involuntary behaviours), adaptive responses (e.g., catching a ball), adaptive skills (e.g., ADL skills), and adaptive patterns (e.g., doing a job). Each step along the continuum involves increasingly complex behaviours. The continuum emphasizes the relationship of adaptive responses to other aspects of human behaviour and offers structure for authentic occupational therapy practice.

---

113. Rogers, J. C. (1982). Order and disorder in medicine and occupational therapy. *Am J Occup Ther, 36*, 29-35.

Keywords: adaptation, biopsychosocial

The author explores the meanings of the three concepts of order, disorder, and change. Differences in orientation to these concepts between occupational therapy and medicine are discussed. It is recommended that occupational therapy use these concepts to develop a generic theory of occupational performance, which does not rely on the medical model.

---

114. Montgomery, M. (1984). Resources of adaptation for daily living: A classification of therapeutic implications for occupational therapy. *Occupational Therapy in Health Care, 1*, 9-24

Keywords: adaptation, environment, hierarchy

Adaptation is defined as flexible behaviour to meet the changing needs of a changing environment. Occupational behaviour thus changes over time as a result of interactions with the environment. Resources for adaptation are those inherent and learned abilities that the individual uses to deal with daily living problems. The author distinguishes three time frames for adaptation: evolution, referring to the inherited central nervous system organisation and processing capabilities; ontogeny, referring to the acquisition and integration of skills over the lifetime; and immediate adaptation, referring to a situation-specific problem-solving process.

---

115. Breines, E. B. (1989). Development, change and continuity theories: An analysis. *Canadian Journal of Occupational Therapy, 56*, 109-112.

Keywords: adaptation, development, hierarchy

An analysis of various developmental theories from other disciplines reveals that most of these theories tend to be stage-descriptive, and Breines condemns them as inconsistent with occupational therapy beliefs. Instead, she suggests that continuity and change are both adaptive and developmental phenomena. She asserts that adaptation is change that happens by degrees in response to the environment and that development is the sum of adaptations.

116. Rosenfeld, M. (1989) Occupational disruption and adaptation: A study of house fire victims. *Am J Occup Ther, 43, 89-96.*

    Keywords: adaptation, process

    Rosenfeld uses the example of house fire victims to study the process of adaptation. She outlined a four-step process consisting of crystallisation of the conflict, recognition of patterns, evaluation of occupational repertoire, and occupational shift.

117. Schkade, J. K., & Schultz, S. (1992). Occupational adaptation: Toward a holistic approach for contemporary practice. Part 2. *Am J Occup Ther, 46, 917-925.*

    Keywords: adaptation, competence, environment

    This is the second of two articles advancing a frame of reference for occupational therapy based on three assumptions: that adaptation occurs in times of transition; that the motivation to adapt is intrinsic; and that occupation is the vehicle for adaptation. Occupational adaptation is, therefore, a process that is nonhierarchical and nonstage-specific, whereby internal and external experiences contribute to functional changes aimed at mastery. Adaptation happens at both conscious and unconscious levels. The article advances a practice model based on the therapeutic environment, the application of occupational activity, and the experience of mastery.

118. Kielhofner, G. (1995). *A model of human occupation: Theory and applications* (2nd ed.). Baltimore: Williams & Wilkins.

    Keywords: adaptation, process

    In this second edition of Kielhofner's book on the model of human occupation, he defines adaptation as a process skill aimed at correcting problems and learning from the consequences of errors that occur in the course of actions. This process includes noticing that a problem exists, modifying either the self or the environment, adjusting to the change, and anticipating the benefits of the adaptation. The performance subsystem is further differentiated into mind, brain, and body components.

119. Frank, G. (1996). The concept of adaptation as a foundation for occupational science research. In R. Zemke & F. Clark (Eds.), *Occupational science: The evolving discipline.* Philadelphia: F. A. Davis.

    Keywords: adaptation, environment, science

    This chapter reviews the concept of adaptation advanced by King and highlights the four principles of adaptive responses: active, response to environment, self-reinforcing, and habitual. She underlines the idea that adaptive responses are nested within adaptive systems. Frank defines adaptation as the process of selecting and organizing occupational responses to improve quality of life in an ever-changing environment.

120. Nelson, D. (1996). Therapeutic occupation: A definition. *Am J Occup Ther, 50,* 775-782.

Keywords: adaptation, competence, terminology

The article focuses on occupation as a therapeutic tool with a special category of occupation. A number of terms are defined, such as occupational synthesis, referring to the design of occupational form based on therapeutic principles. Nelson suggests that the developmental structure of an individual is composed of both physical maturation and occupational adaptation. Occupational adaptation is defined as the positive effects of occupational performance, leading either to the restoration of previously lost abilities or the acquisition of new ones.

121. Spencer, J. C., Davidson, H. A., & White, V. K. (1996). Continuity and change: Past experience as adaptive repertoire in occupational adaptation. *Am J Occup Ther, 50,* 526-534.

Keywords: adaptation, systems, time

Spencer and colleagues look at changes in the life narrative and attempt to explain how people maintain continuity and integrity of the self in the midst of change. They define adaptation as a cumulative, interactive process between the organism and the environment, whereby genetic and cultural processes from the past are integrated with environmental demands in the present to enhance the adaptive repertoire for the future. This process involves appraisal of the situation and the existing adaptive repertoire, reconfiguration of old behaviours, and assimilation of new skills into the repertoire.

122. Schultz, S., & Schkade, J. (1997). Adaptation. In C. Christiansen & C. Baum (Eds.), *Occupational therapy: Enabling function and well-being* (2nd ed., pp. 458-481). Thorofare, NJ: SLACK Incorporated.

Keywords: adaptation, process, values

This very comprehensive chapter reviews the history of the concept of adaptation and its importance in the development of occupational therapy. It offers 10 beliefs about adaptation that are central to its role in occupational therapy, dealing with person-environment fit, level of adaptation, importance of mastery, and its relationship to well-being. It concludes with a review of the occupational adaptation process.

123. Jonsson, A. T., Moller, A., & Brimby, G. (1999). Managing occupations in everyday life to achieve adaptation. *Am J Occup Ther, 53,* 353-362.

Keywords: adaptation, coping

This article acknowledges that adaptation is a concept that is pervasive in the theory of many disciplines. The authors define adaptation according to coping theory, as a process through which an individual maintains an acceptable compromise in relationships with the environment. They recognize that disability limits the adaptive repertoire, and that adaptive resources can be acquired in three ways: through evolution, development, and learning.

ACCOMMODATION

124. **Jongbloed, L. (1990). A new definition of disability: Implications for rehabilitation practice and social policy.** *Canadian Journal of Occupational Therapy, 57, 32-38.*

Keywords: accommodation, disability, environment

The paper examines the impact of a socio-political definition of disability on the roles of rehabilitation practitioners. The definition places the responsibility for disability on the environment and requires alteration in the physical and social environment.

125. **Crist, P. (1992). The Americans with Disabilities Act of 1990 and employees with mental impairments: Personal efficacy.** *Am J Occup Ther, 46, 434-443.*

Keywords: accommodation, disability, environment

The paper discusses the role of occupational therapy relative to people with mental illness in upholding the terms of the Americans with Disabilities Act (ADA) in the United States. It deals with four aspects of the environment and the potential need for accommodation.

126. **Bachelder, J., & List Hilton, C. (1994). Implications of the Americans with Disabilities Act of 1990 for elderly persons.** *Am J Occup Ther, 48, 73-81.*

Keywords: accommodation, disability, environment

This paper applies the provisions of the ADA to the needs of older people relative to workplace and community accessibility. The authors emphasize the elimination of structural and programmatic barriers and accommodation for functional and sensory losses.

127. **Mutchnick, I., & Blount, M. L. (1996). A pilot study on attitudes toward making reasonable accommodations for occupational therapists with disabilities.** *Occupational Therapy International, 3, 49-66.*

Keywords: accommodation, disability, values

This small study investigated attitudes and knowledge of the ADA provisions in regards to the employment of occupational therapists. Those who had received training on the provisions of the Act had more positive attitudes toward accommodations than those who had not.

---

128. Scott, P. (1996). Employment for individuals with mental disabilities: ADA unlocked the door but who has the handle? *Occupational Therapy in Mental Health, 10,* 49-64.

Keywords: accommodation, disability, work

The author discusses the issue of the necessity to disclose invisible disability, such as mental illness, in order to receive accommodation under the ADA. The role of occupational therapy is highlighted in terms of preparing both clients and employers to undergo accommodation.

---

129. Hemmingsson, H., & Borell, L. (2000). Accommodation needs and student-environment fit in upper secondary schools for students with severe disabilities. *Canadian Journal of Occupational Therapy, 67,* 162-172.

Keywords: accommodation, disability, environment

The article discusses needs for physical and social accommodation of high school students with disabilities. Accommodations on general, group, and individual levels are discussed, with attention to both curricular and extra-curricular activities.

---

130. Dyck, I., & Jongbloed, L. (2000). Women with multiple sclerosis and employment issues: A focus on social and institutional environments. *Canadian Journal of Occupational Therapy, 67,* 337-346.

Keywords: accommodation, disability, work

This study of women with MS shows that employment status was affected by employer attitudes, work conditions, and family support, as well as the individual's functional status. It highlights the importance of social and institutional factors in shaping occupational performance.

9

THE PHYSICAL DETERMINANTS OF OCCUPATION

Debra Stewart, MSc

Introduction

The physical area of occupational therapy theory deals with the physical components of occupation, task, and activity. The articles referred to below all contribute to our understanding of occupation as an issue of physical function, primarily determined by physical capabilities or disabilities. This theory area includes concepts from biomechanics, kinetics, energy conservation, orthotics, and prosthetics. The physical rehabilitative approach has a strong basis in the physical sciences, such as anatomy, physiology, and kinesiology.

A Brief History of Theory of the Physical Determinants of Occupation

The early literature in this area describes a shift away from the origins of occupational therapy in the area of mental health. It starts near the end of World War I, in response to the needs of returning veterans, many of whom had amputations. Developments in automation and urban industrialization also resulted in physical disabilities from industrial and motor accidents. With the emergence of the biomedical model in the 1920s, physical rehabilitation became stronger. Activity analysis, graduated exercise, and prevocational training were specific areas of occupational therapy practice described in articles through the 1930s.

World War II also had a strong influence on the emerging field of physical rehabilitation and occupational therapy. With an increase in the prevalence of physical disability and chronic conditions, the scope of practice of occupational therapy broadened. The literature demonstrates this evolution, with more physical treatment techniques emerging and an increase in the use of prosthetic and orthotic technology. As medical science advanced, the occupational therapy literature about physical function and dysfunction in the 1950s and 1960s focused on techniques rather than theory. Specific treatment areas included kinetics, orthotics, self-help, adaptive devices and techniques, work evaluation and retraining, and grading activity to promote physical function.

The 1970s and 1980s saw a shift in the literature with a call for more emphasis on theory, rather than techniques. There was very little written about physical rehabilitative theory in these two decades, and it was noted that few theoretical models in occupational therapy were based on biomechanical concepts alone. The role of the occupational therapist appeared to be moving beyond the assessment and treatment of physical skills alone to view the whole person in context of his or her daily environments and occupations. The goals of occupational therapy in the area of physical disability were moving to independence and quality of life, rather than focusing strictly on performance components, such as endurance, range of motion, and strength. This evolution continued through the 1990s, with literature demonstrating occupational therapy practice broadening into areas of leisure and sexuality, sport and recreation, as well as the traditional areas of vocational rehabilitation, equipment, and activity adaptation.

KEYWORDS USED IN THIS CHAPTER

Activity	Environment	Leisure	Sexuality
Assistive devices	Exercise	Models	Strength
Beliefs	History	Modalities	Work
Biomechanical	Independence	Motivation	
Competence	Identity	Range of motion	
Endurance	Kinesiology	Rehabilitation	

Bibliographic Entries for the Physical Determinants of Occupation

131. Pedretti, L. W. (1981). *Occupational therapy: Practice skills for physical disabilities.* **St. Louis, MO: C. V. Mosby.**

Keywords: biomechanical, disability, models

This is a basic comprehensive textbook for occupational therapists working with people with physical disabilities. (see 4th edition; reference #159)

132. Rogers, J. C. (1982). The spirit of independence: The evolution of a philosophy. *Am J Occup Ther, 36,* 709-715.

Keywords: beliefs, environment, independence

The author reviews the history of occupational therapy philosophy to explain the significance of our beliefs about functional independence. Current beliefs are articulated and implications for practice are explored. Three key concepts related to functional independence are discussed in detail: (1) personal components of independent behaviour, (2) the environment, and (3) the person-environment interaction.

133. **Ben-Shlomo, L. S. (1983). The effect of physical exercise on self-attitudes.** *Occupational Therapy in Mental Health, 3,* 11-28.

Keywords: exercise, identity

This article reviews the research on the effect of physical exercise on self-attitudes of those within a rehabilitation group and a nonrehabilitation group. The findings suggest that physical exercise enhances self-attitudes in individuals with physical and/or emotional disabilities. However, for those without these disabilities, self-attitude enhancement depends on their initial physical-emotional condition, their personality, and the exercise program itself.

134. **Trombly, C. A., & Quintana, L. A. (1983). Activity analysis: Electromyographic and electrogoniometric verification.** *Occupational Therapy Journal of Research, 3,* 104-120.

Keywords: activity, range of motion, strength

A study was conducted to document extrinsic finger muscle function and interaction during five exercises that resembled activities commonly used in occupational therapy. Electromyographic and electrogoniometric techniques were used to identify factors to consider in activity analysis.

135. **Klein, M. M. (1984). The therapeutics of recreation.** *Physical and Occupational Therapy in Paediatrics, 4,* 9-11.

Keywords: activity, leisure

Sport and recreation are viewed as tools that therapists can use for rehabilitation and education. When combined with therapeutic needs, they can become an enjoyable and exciting means to the long-term goal of enhanced quality of life. Several examples of integrating therapeutic needs with sport and recreation for people with physical disabilities are provided.

136. **LeVeau, B. F. (1984). Team sports.** *Physical and Occupational Therapy in Paediatrics, 4,* 65-75.

Keywords: activity, leisure, motivation

Team games are considered to be important for a child with a disability, as they allow the child to be a contributing group member. The needs and motivational drives of children with and without disabilities can be met through participation in team sports. It is recommended that children with disabilities participate on regular teams without modifications; but when necessary, modifications can be made to rules, equipment, and facilities. The attitude and role of the team leaders is viewed as critical to the success of this integration.

137. Reed, K. L. (1984). Descriptive models: Sensorimotor and cognitive performance areas. In K. L. Reed (Ed.), *Models of practice in occupational therapy* (pp. 278-364). Baltimore: Williams & Wilkins.

Keywords: biomechanical, models

In this chapter, three biomechanical models are described: Baldwin's reconstruction model, Taylor's orthopedic model, and Licht's kinetic model. Each model is described in terms of its frame of reference and assumptions, important concepts and expected results, and assessment instruments and intervention strategies. An analysis and critique of the biomechanical models is also provided.

138. Brintnell, E. S., Cardwell, M. T., Robinson, I. M., & Madill, H. M. (1986). The rehabilitation era: Friend or foe. *Canadian Journal of Occupational Therapy, 53,* 27-33.

Keyword: rehabilitation

This article reviews three key articles written in the 1950s and 1960s about occupational therapy that capture the trends of the period. The focus of that period was rehabilitation, and with it there was an increase in demand for occupational therapy services. Conclusions are drawn about the "mixed blessings" of the rehabilitation movement for occupational therapy.

139. Hoyle Parent, L. (1986). Energy: The illusive factor in daily activity. *Occupational Therapy in Health Care, 3,* 5-15.

Keywords: endurance, exercise

This article focuses on people with energy deficiencies, and the role of occupational therapy in planning treatment programs that involve diverse amounts of energy use by those patients. The author suggests the use of exercise and reflex movement patterns as a means by which energy conservation can be accomplished. The psychosocial aspects of intervening with people with energy deficiencies are also discussed.

140. Bonum, H. S., & Rogers, J. C. (1987). The use and effectiveness of assistive devices possessed by patients seen within home care. *Occupational Therapy Journal of Research, 7*(3), 181-191.

Keywords: assistive devices, rehabilitation

This study explores the effectiveness and use of 54 assistive devices belonging to 30 clients who received home care. The article discusses the types of devices used and the frequency of use. It is concluded that the majority of these devices were effective. Reasons for nonuse are also discussed.

141. **Kennedy, M. (1987). Occupational therapists as sexual rehabilitation professionals using the physical rehabilitative frame of reference. *Canadian Journal of Occupational Therapy, 54,* 189-193.**

   Keywords: rehabilitation, sexuality

   The physical rehabilitative frame of reference is presented as a useful model to assist physically disabled adults in adjusting to changes in their sexual activities. This frame of reference provides theoretical justification for the role of occupational therapists in the area of leisure skills. The role of the occupational therapist is viewed as providing information on sexual activities to physically disabled adults.

142. **MacNeela, J. C. (1987). An overview of therapeutic positioning for multiply-handicapped persons, including augmentative communication users. *Physical and Occupational Therapy in Paediatrics, 7,* 60.**

   Keyword: assistive devices

   This article provides therapists with a review of the literature related to formal studies and guidelines for the use of therapeutic positioning and adaptive equipment for clients with multiple physical needs. General principles for clinical implementation of therapeutic positioning are discussed, with specific examples related to the use of augmentative communication devices.

143. **McGrain, P., & Hague, M. A. (1987). An electromyographic study of the middle deltoid and middle trapezius muscles during warping. *Occupational Therapy Journal of Research, 7,* 225-233.**

   Keywords: activity, exercise, strength

   This study examines the relationship between horizontal and vertical placement of a warping board (used in weaving), and the amounts of myoelectric activity elicited in the middle deltoid and middle trapezius. This study has implications for occupational therapy because therapeutic exercise and its uses are considered to be important in occupational therapy.

144. **McKenna, K. T., & Maas, F. (1987). Mean and peak heart rate predication using estimated energy costs of jobs. *Occupational Therapy Journal of Research, 7,* 323-334.**

   Keywords: endurance, exercise, work

   The measurement of heart rate is advocated as an effective and sensitive measure of exertion and activity intensity for job analysis. The authors, therefore, studied hospital employees in a variety of different work conditions to provide normative information on the heart rate or exertion level of a number of hospital jobs.

145. Schkade, J. K., Feibelman, A., & Cook, J. D. (1987). Occupational potential in a population with Duchenne muscular dystrophy. *Occupational Therapy Journal of Research, 7*, 289-300.

Keywords: competence, endurance, strength

Occupational potential was assessed in 25 males, ages 7 to 23, with Duchenne muscular dystrophy. Standardized tests were used to examine sensory deficits, strength, fatigue, and endurance. Occupational therapy is concerned with this area of study because clients, especially adolescents, tend to become passive and unmotivated as the disease progresses, having no occupational roles and, therefore, no feelings of competence.

146. Kennedy, M. (1988). Application of pressure: A principle in the biomechanical frame of reference. *Canadian Journal of Occupational Therapy, 55*(1), 31-33.

Keywords: biomechanical, range of motion

The author proposes the addition of the principle of pressure application to the biomechanical frame of reference to assist occupational therapists in more appropriately assessing the need for application of pressure as a means of preventing deterioration in range of motion.

147. Thibodeaux, C., & Ludwig, F. M. (1988). Intrinsic motivation in product-oriented and non-product-oriented activities. *Am J Occup Ther, 42*, 169-175.

Keywords: activity, endurance, motivation

Purposeful activity is defined as one of the primary modalities of occupational therapy. This article discusses the results of a study that examined purposeful activity as an intrinsic motivator. The two activities selected for the study were sanding a cutting board that subjects were told they could keep and sanding a piece of wood that they could not keep. The dependent variables were the effort exerted and the time spent in sanding.

148. Short-DeGraff, M. A., & Healey, S. M. (1989). Exercise and activity in the promotion of health: An annotated bibliography. *Occupational Therapy in Health Care, 5*, 69-85.

Keywords: activity, exercise

The potential benefits of exercise on physical and mental health are explored in this annotated bibliography. The article aims to provide occupational therapists with a resource to become aware of the present status of exercise-related research.

149. **Creighton, C. (1992). The origin and evolution of activity analysis.** *Am J Occup Ther, 46,* 45-48.

Keywords: activity, history

The history of activity analysis from World War I to the present is described in this article. The most systematic early use of activity analysis was in occupational therapy for physical dysfunction, particularly in military hospitals. Development of the concept was gradual until the 1970s, when the delineation of theoretical frames of reference for practice led to important changes. Today, activity analysis is viewed as a multifaceted process that involves both generic and specific components.

150. **Hagedorn, R. (1992). Frames of reference. In R. Hagedorn (Ed.),** *Occupational therapy: Foundations for practice—Models, frames of reference, and core skills* **(pp. 17-39). Edinburgh, Scotland: Churchill Livingstone.**

Keywords: biomechanical, models

In this chapter, the author describes five different frames of reference and their general approaches, including the physiological frame of reference. The biomechanical approach is contrasted with the neurodevelopmental approach, as both are considered part of the physiological frame of reference. A brief summary of the assumptions, patient-therapist relationship, examples of application and techniques, and advantages and disadvantages of the biomechanical approach are given.

151. **Kielhofner, G. (1992). The biomechanical model. In G. Kielhofner (Ed.),** *Conceptual foundations of occupational therapy* **(1st ed., pp. 91-106). Philadelphia: F. A. Davis.**

Keywords: biomechanical, models

The biomechanical model is discussed in terms of its focus and interdisciplinary base. The author also provides a description and summary of the theory underlying therapeutic interventions guided by this model, and the approaches and methods of assessments and interventions. Further research in this area, applicable to occupation, is recommended.

152. **Mathiowetz, V. (1993). Role of physical performance component evaluations in occupational therapy functional assessment.** *Am J Occup Ther, 47,* 225-230.

Keywords: history, range of motion, strength

The history of physical performance component (PPC) evaluations, including strength and range of motion, is reviewed. Changes within and outside the profession of occupational therapy are supporting a move to focus assessment more on occupation and role performance, while PPC evaluation should shift to a secondary role. Although PPC evaluations may be less prominent than in the past, they will continue to play an important role in occupational therapy practice and research.

153. Bailey, D. M. (1994). Technology for adults with multiple impairments: A trilogy of reports. *Am J Occup Ther, 48,* 341-345.

Keywords: assistive devices, endurance

This article describes three case studies of clients using powered assistive devices. The findings support the tenets of client enthusiasm, responsiveness, and stamina that are used in occupational therapy to help a client achieve success in using assistive technology.

154. Smith, R. (1995). A client-centred model for equipment prescription. *Occupational Therapy in Health Care, 9*(4), 39-52.

Keyword: assistive devices

The author reviews studies of individuals with physical dysfunction that suggest that clients often fail to use equipment because the therapist's equipment prescription focuses exclusively on the physical aspects of treatment. A client-centred model for equipment prescription is then outlined, and a case study of an individual with a spinal cord injury is presented to illustrate the application of this model.

155. Dutton, R. (Ed.). (1995). *Clinical reasoning in physical disabilities.* Baltimore: Williams & Wilkins.

Keywords: biomechanical, models, rehabilitation

This textbook offers a through summary of the biomechanical and physical rehabilitative approaches to therapy using detailed explanations of the clinical reasoning processes for each.

156. Trombly, C. A. (1995). Theoretical foundations for practice. In C. A. Trombly (Ed.), *Occupational therapy for physical dysfunction* (4th ed., pp. 15-27). Baltimore: Williams & Wilkins.

Keywords: biomechanical, models, rehabilitation

The author describes the hierarchical model that guides occupational therapy for physical dysfunction and five major conceptual models of practice. Physical rehabilitative models described include the biomechanical and rehabilitative models.

157. Exner, C. E. (1996). Development of hand skills. In J. Case-Smith, A. S. Allen, & P. N. Pratt (Eds.), *Occupational therapy for children* (3rd ed., pp. 268-306). St. Louis, MO: C. V. Mosby.

Keywords: biomechanical, children

The author describes the components of hand skills, factors that influence hand skills, and the relationship between hand skills and function performance in play, self-care, and school. The biomechanical frame of reference is discussed briefly as one of six commonly used frames of reference in the assessments and interventions described in this chapter for children with hand skill problems.

158. Hinojosa, J., Kramer, P., & Nuse, P. N. (1996). Foundations of practice: Developmental principles, theories, and frames of reference. In J. Case-Smith, A. S. Allen, & P. N. Pratt (Eds.), *Occupational therapy for children* (3rd ed., pp. 25-45). St. Louis, MO: C. V. Mosby.

Keywords: biomechanical, children

In this chapter, the authors describe the major developmental theories and principles that underlie the nine frames of reference frequently used in occupational therapy, which are highlighted. The biomechanical frame of reference is briefly described in this chapter and is employed when a person has musculoskeletal or neuromuscular dysfunction.

159. Pedretti, L. W., & Zoltan, B. (1996). *Occupational therapy: Practice skills for physical disability* (4th ed.). St. Louis, MO: C. V. Mosby.

Keywords: biomechanical, disability, models

This is the fourth edition of this comprehensive textbook on physical disability. It offers chapters on both the disabilities themselves and the occupational therapy approaches to treatment of physical disability.

160. Kielhofner, G. (1997). Biomechanical model. In G. Kielhofner (Ed.), *Conceptual foundations of occupational therapy* (2nd ed., pp. 109-125). Philadelphia: F. A. Davis.

Keywords: biomechanical, models

The biomechanical model is briefly described in terms of its applications and interdisciplinary base. Theoretical arguments underlying order and dysfunction are also discussed, and three therapeutic approaches are presented. Five methods of application are described, and the author highlights suggestions for further research.

161. McGuire, M. (1997). Physical agent modalities: Position paper. *Am J Occup Ther, 51*(10), 870-871.

Keywords: activity, modalities

This paper clarifies the parameters for the appropriate use of physical agent modalities in occupational therapy practice. These modalities are defined and described. The theoretical and technical education necessary for safe and appropriate use of any physical agent modality is suggested.

162. Minor, M. A. (1997). Promoting health and physical fitness. In C. Christiansen & C. Baum (Eds.), *Occupational therapy: Enabling function and well-being* (2nd ed., pp. 254-287). Thorofare, NJ: SLACK Incorporated.

Keywords: endurance, range of motion, rehabilitation, strength

The author discusses the concept of physical fitness as a framework in the rehabilitation and study of human performance. Five major components of physical fitness, cardiorespiratory function, muscle strength, endurance, flexibility, and body composition are discussed. Methods of assessment and prescription of exercise and activity to promote physical fitness and positive adaptations are discussed, and several factors affecting performance are presented.

163. **Dutton, R. (1998). Biomechanical frame of reference. In M. E. Neistadt, & E. B. Crepeau (Eds.), *Willard & Spackman's occupational therapy* (9th ed., pp. 540-542). Philadelphia: Lippincott Raven.**

Keywords: biomechanical, models

In this chapter, the assumptions and six domains of concern of the biomechanical frame of reference are highlighted. Evaluation methods and the effects of using this frame of reference on client-practitioner interactions are described in view of the current emphasis on functional outcomes. The strengths and limitations of this approach are discussed, and recommendations for research into the relationship between biomechanical gains and functional outcomes are made.

164. **Friedland J. (1998). Looking back. Occupational therapy and rehabilitation: An awkward alliance. *Am J Occup Ther*, 52(5): 373-380.**

Keywords: history, rehabilitation

This article argues that although occupational therapy and rehabilitation are often considered synonymous, the latter is but one aspect of the former. Early influences on occupational therapy are briefly reviewed, and some philosophical ideas about activity are described. The article demonstrates that the origins of occupational therapy and rehabilitation had little in common. Although current definitions of rehabilitation offer an appropriate fit for occupational therapy, rehabilitation continues to see engagement in occupations as a separate and subsequent step. The article concludes by considering future directions.

165. **Reed, K. L., & Sanderson, S. N. (1999). Models currently in practice. In K. L. Reed, & S. N. Sanderson (Eds.), *Concepts of occupational therapy* (4th ed., pp. 238-263). Baltimore: Lippincott Williams & Wilkins.**

Keywords: biomechanical, models

In this chapter, the biomechanical model is described in terms of its frame of reference, assumptions, concepts, assessments, planning, and intervention. A critical analysis of the model is also provided.

166. Bracciano, A. G. (Ed.). (2000). *Physical agent modalities: Theory and application for the occupational therapist.* Thorofare, NJ: SLACK Incorporated.

Keywords: activities, biomechanical, modalities

This textbook focuses on the use of physical agent modalities in occupational therapy. Basic principles and theories, biophysical underpinnings, and clinical decision-making issues are part of each chapter.

SOME IMPORTANT IDEAS ABOUT THE PHYSICAL DETERMINANTS OF OCCUPATION:

- Occupational performance problems originating in the musculoskeletal system can be understood using theory in this area.
- This theory area pertains to problems caused by deficits in the physical performance area.
- This area of theory locates the source of occupational performance problems in the person.
- The main physical determinants of occupation are strength, range of motion, and endurance.
- Occupations and activities can be graded to remediate strength, range of motion, and endurance.
- Occupational conceptual models help us to understand the physical requirements of self-care, productivity, and leisure.
- Manual muscle testing, goniometry, and activity tolerance are typical assessments belonging to the basic model of practice for this theory area.
- Activity analysis for physical requirements is an important part of the occupational model of practice in this area.
- Biomechanical and rehabilitative are two named theories in this theory area.
- The use of splints and adaptive aids to replace physical function is part of the occupational model of practice in this area.
- Energy conservation, work simplification, and joint protection are all part of the occupational model of practice in this area.
- This theory area is rich in history, dating from the period following World War I.

FOLLOWING IS A PRACTICAL PROBLEM THAT MAY HELP TO RAISE SOME
OF THE IMPORTANT IDEAS IN THE AREA OF PHYSICAL DETERMINANTS
OF OCCUPATION:

Dave is an occupational therapist who works in the area of orthopaedics and rheumatology. He has been seeing Mrs. Dixon once a week as an outpatient. Mrs. Dixon is 36 years old and has rheumatoid arthritis. She has been receiving therapy intermittently since her first acute exacerbation of arthritis some years ago. The main joints involved are in her hands, shoulders, and lower back. She has tried a number of different splints during this time but only wears resting splints at night now. Mrs. Dixon is a legal secretary in a small law firm. She has two children, 10 and 12 years old, and her husband is a grocery store manager. Recently, Mrs. Dixon was again referred to outpatient OT following an acute period of about 6 weeks.

After carefully assessing Mrs. Dixon with a variety of occupational therapy assessments of physical functioning, Dave began a program aimed at:

1. Building up strength, while being attentive to the potential for further damage and deformity

2. Increasing Mrs. Dixon's tolerance for activity

3. Examining her daily routines for work simplification, energy conservation, compensatory techniques, and the use of adaptive equipment.

Mrs. Dixon has considerable enthusiasm for the first two goals, as this is what she believes rehabilitation to be about. But she becomes impatient and agitated when Dave suggests that there are some activities that she will simply not be able to do anymore or will have to do in different ways. Dave is becoming increasingly frustrated with Mrs. Dixon's "unrealistic expectations" of therapy and her unwillingness to consider compensatory techniques. Dave realizes that he needs to be able to explain to Mrs. Dixon his rationale for all three therapy goals. He, therefore, consults his knowledge base in the area of physical rehabilitation for occupational therapy concepts and principles that will help to explain to Mrs. Dixon what he is doing and why.

THE PSYCHOLOGICAL-EMOTIONAL DETERMINANTS OF OCCUPATION

10

Terry Krupa, PhD

Introduction

Psychoemotional theory, or theory about the psychological and emotional determinants of occupation, provides a framework for understanding why and how human beings are inherently motivated toward successful engagement in self-care, leisure, and productivity. It explains the occupational nature of humans and provides important information about the processes through which occupation can be enhanced.

According to the tenets of psychoemotional theory, individuals are motivated to participate in occupation to meet dynamic needs that are elicited by both internal and environmental factors. In addition to basic physiological needs, humans engage in occupations that satisfy psychoemotional needs that promote growth, belonging, and self-actualization. All of these needs are fundamental to survival. Engagement in occupation is believed to promote the levels of competence and autonomy necessary for humans to adapt to their ever-changing environments.

Human occupations are so complex as to allow for an almost seamless satisfaction of multiple needs simultaneously. For example, the self-care activity of preparing a meal might be constructed to eliminate hunger, fulfill belonging needs, and allow for self-expression. This feature of occupation makes it a particularly powerful therapeutic tool.

The idea of *self* is a central construct in psychoemotional theory. The self integrates all of the elements of the individual to constitute a distinct identity. It helps us to understand why individuals engage in particular occupations and activities. Along with motivation, other psychoemotional factors associated with the self include attitudes, interests, beliefs, awareness and experience, self-concept, sexuality, empowerment, self-efficacy, personal causation, self-determination, and sense of competence. The nature of an individual's participation in occupation is an expression of the self, and occupation is subsequently imbued with personal meaning. The exploration of personal meaning is an important component of holistic occupational therapy practice.

In psychoemotional theory, the individual's thoughts and feelings are believed to influence occupational performance. Specifically, the focus is on the extent to which an individual's thoughts and feelings reflect realistic appraisals of the self and the self within the larger world, thereby enabling initiation and direction of successful occupational behaviours. In turn, engaging in occupations promotes personal growth and provides the individual with important feedback about the self as unique and competent.

Specific disorders can directly disturb thoughts and feelings in a manner that disrupts occupation. For example, psychosis can disrupt the stability of thoughts and feelings necessary for a stable self-identity, and it can impair the ability to accurately interpret the broader environment. Disturbances in thoughts and feelings may occur secondary to other health-related problems. For example, depression associated with a pervasive physical illness can dampen an individual's interest for everyday occupations. Finally, occupation itself can influence thoughts and feelings. Unemployment, for example, has been associated with weakening the initiative for activity by undermining personal causation and sense of competence.

Coping, or the individual's adaptation to environmental demands and challenges, also falls under the purview of psychoemotional theory. Coping relies on both the individual's appraisal of the demands and potential threats of a situation, and on the individual's efforts to use available personal resources to manage the situation.

A Brief History of Psychoemotional Theory

The beginnings of occupational therapy in the early 20th century were focused primarily on the treatment of mental disorders. The early champions of occupational therapy recognized that ill-balanced occupation could elicit mental disturbances. They developed the idea that engagement in occupation had curative properties, particularly through its potential to place limits on introspection, replace gloomy and unwholesome thoughts and feelings, and induce self-reliance, mastery, and psychic energy.

The approach to occupations in these early times was prescriptive. There was an effort to match occupations to individual dispositions and temperaments. The motivating aspects of occupation were considered to ensure therapeutic benefits, although in practice this was constrained by the institutional context of treatment.

The return of veterans from World War I demonstrated the relationship between psychological and emotional issues in physical disability. Occupational therapy practices were implemented with veterans with disabilities, both to restore mental health and emotional well-being and to promote the volitional properties of activity to sustain effort for physical remediation. It also marked the beginning of an appreciation for the relationship between the personal meaning of occupation and its meaning in a broader social context.

The psychoanalytical theories proposed by Freud and his followers had a profound influence on the development of psychoemotional theory in occupational therapy. While the influence of analytic theories appears as early as the 1930s, they gained prominence in the 1950s and 1960s. These early analytic theories highlighted the influence of intrapsychic factors on occupational behaviour, the expression of intrapsychic content through occupations, and the use of occupations to enable the reconciliation of intrapsychic conflicts to positively influence adaptation.

Early psychoanalytic theories in occupational therapy tended to be highly reductionistic, focusing on psychological and emotional aspects of the individual rather than on occupation. When the profession became more focused on occupation in the 1970s, several important ideas and assumptions underlying analytic theory evolved and were integrated into occupational therapy theory. These included such important concepts as self, as well as object relations and specific occupational therapy interventions such as the therapeutic use of self, therapeutic milieu, projective techniques, and the therapeutic use of groups.

Occupational therapy's understanding of the factors associated with the motivational properties of occupation was influenced by the development of psychological theories of motivation in the 1960s. These theories provided a foundation for the understanding of both intrinsic and extrinsic motivation, enabling the development of such important concepts as sense of competence and the drive for mastery. The ideas underlying these psychological theories were applied in occupational therapy to understand the motivational issues associated with a broad spectrum of disabilities.

In the 1960s occupational therapy witnessed the beginnings of the application of behavioural theories. Behavioural theories provided a basis for understanding and influencing performance in relation to the objective behaviours and skills of occupation. The processes and principles of learning were integrated into occupational therapy practice. With its focus on the objective aspects of human behaviour, the behaviour therapies were particularly attractive to occupational therapy as the profession began to address issues of accountability and outcome measurement.

In the 1970s and 1980s, behavioural theories evolved to include a focus on behaviour in interaction with thoughts and affect. These cognitive behavioural theories were applied in structured programs in occupational therapy to improve occupational performance and psychological well-being. Cognitive behavioural approaches engaged individuals in actively reflecting and acting on their own thoughts and feelings in relation to desired goals. These approaches were a precursor to the contemporary applications of psychoemotional theory that address the experience of occupation, the personal processes of empowerment, and the construction of self-identity through occupation.

KEYWORDS USED IN THIS CHAPTER

Activity	Coping	Locus of control	Psychoeducational
Adolescent	Disability	Meaning	Psychological
Affect	Emotion	Models	Self
Aging	Empowerment	Motivation	Sexuality
Behavioural	Groups	Personal causation	Stress
Cognition	Hope	Phenomenology	Values
Cognitive	Humanism	Play	Volition
behavoural	Identity	Psychodynamic	Work
Competence			

Bibliographic Entries for Psychological-Emotional Determinants of Occupation

167. Bell, C. H. (1975). Competition as motivation incentive. *Am J Occup Ther, 29*, 277-279.

Keywords: activity, motivation

The author proposes that competition may motivate individuals to achieve occupational therapy objectives. Risk taking is suggested as an indicator of competitiveness.

168. Jodrell, R. D., & Sanson-Fisher, R. (1975). Basic concepts of behavior therapy: An experiment involving disturbed adolescent girls. *Am J Occup Ther, 29,* 620-624.

Keywords: adolescent, behaviour

This article illustrates the application of behaviour therapy principles and techniques. The behavioural approach is applied in teaching social skills for community adjustment to adolescent girls with behavioural disturbances.

169. Perem, L., & Renwick, R. (1975). Use of three techniques in an insight group. *Canadian Journal of Occupational Therapy, 42,* 49-53.

Keywords: group, self

This article describes group techniques for heightening the development of openness and self-awareness.

170. Norman, C. (1976). Behavior modification: A perspective. *Am J Occup Ther, 30,* 491-497.

Keyword: behaviour

This article describes the process of behaviour change using behaviour modification principles.

171. Burke, J. P. (1977). A clinical perspective on motivation: Pawn versus origin. *Am J Occup Ther, 31,* 254-258.

Keywords: motivation, personal causation

This article presents personal causation as an integral factor in human motivation. The principle of active engagement, by matching clients' needs and interests to occupation, motivates human performance in treatment.

172. Magill, J., & Vargo, J. W. (1977). Helplessness, hope and the occupational therapist. *Canadian Journal of Occupational Therapy, 44,* 65-69.

Keywords: personal causation, hope

This article focuses on how personal loss of control can result in mental health decline. Occupational therapy can facilitate hopefulness by re-establishing a sense of control.

173. Hindmarsh, W. A. (1979). Play diagnosis and play therapy. *Am J Occup Ther, 33,* 770-775.

    Keywords: emotion, play, therapeutic relationship

    Play therapy is presented as an approach that allows for the opportunity for the expression of aggression and anger, for a supportive therapeutic relationship, and for exploration and social development.

174. Fidler, G. S. (1981). From crafts to competence. *Am J Occup Ther, 35,* 567-573.

    Keywords: activity, competence

    This article discusses the influence of participation in purposeful activity and the development of the sense of competence.

175. King, N. (1981). Childhood asthma. Part 1: Physiological and psychological aspects. *Australian Occupational Therapy Journal, 28,* 49-54.

176. King, N. (1981). Childhood asthma. Part 2: Recent developments in psychological treatment. *Australian Occupational Therapy Journal, 28,* 101-109.

    Keywords: behavioural, psychological

    In this two-part paper, the author reviews the literature concerning the psychological aspects of childhood asthma and discusses the application of learning behavioural and psychoanalytical theory as the basis for intervention.

177. Burton, J. (1982). Programming to meet the needs of the elderly in institutions. Part 2. *Canadian Journal of Occupational Therapy, 49,* 89-91.

    Keyword: psychological

    Burton develops the idea that the self-actualization process in the elderly institutionalized population can be facilitated through occupational therapy.

178. Lillie, M. D., & Armstrong, H. E. (1982). Contributions to the development of psychoeducational approaches to mental health services. *Am J Occup Ther, 36*(7), 438-443.

    Keywords: cognitive-behavioural, psychoeducational

    This article presents the underlying theory of the psychoeducational approach as applied to an occupational therapy life skills program to improve the occupational skills of people with mental illness.

179. Maslen, D. (1982). Rehabilitation training for community living skills: Concepts and techniques. *Occupational Therapy in Mental Health, 2*, 33-49.

Keyword: behavioural

The author contends that accountability and quality assurance in occupational therapy are facilitated by the use of a behavioural framework to specify outcomes and learning methods related to the acquisition of functional learning skills.

180. Nelson, D. L., Thompson, G., & Moore, J. A. (1982). Identification of factors of affective meaning in four selected activities. *Am J Occup Ther, 36*, 381-387.

Keywords: activity, affect, meaning

This study examined the possibility that activities can be quantified according to affective meaning. Specific affective dimensions included evaluation, power, and activity or action.

181. Stein, F. (1982). A current review of the behavioural frame of reference and its application to occupational therapy. *Occupational Therapy in Mental Health, 2*(4), 35-62.

Keyword: behavioural

In this article, Stein reviews behavioural theory and provides an application of behavioural concepts to occupational therapy. There is a particular focus on social skills training.

182. Teitelman, J. (1982). Eliminating learned helplessness in older rehabilitation patients. *Physical and Occupational Therapy in Geriatrics, 1*, 3-10.

Keywords: aging, motivation

Teitelman discusses the learned helplessness as a theory for understanding the motivational and other psychological and emotional deficits affecting the elderly rehabilitation client.

183. Zemke, R. (1982). The role of theory: Erikson and occupational therapy. *Occupational Therapy in Mental Health, 2*, 45-64.

Keywords: identity, psychological

In this article, Erikson's theory of the development of ego identity is presented as a framework for occupational therapists to understand adjustment to dysfunction.

184. Carter, B. A., Nelson, D. L., & Duncombe, L. W. (1983). The effect of psychological type on the mood and meaning of two collage activities. *Am J Occup Ther, 37,* 688-693.

Keywords: activity, affect, meaning

This study explored the relationship between the perceptual processes of distinct personality types and the affective meanings of activities.

185. Hills-Maguire, G. (1983). An exploratory study of the relationships of valued activities to the life satisfaction of elderly persons. *Occupational Therapy Journal of Research, 3,* 164-172.

Keywords: activity, aging, meaning

This study, focusing on a sample of elderly persons, provided support for the assumption that valued activities are positively related to life satisfaction.

186. Kaplan, K., Mendelson, L. B., & Dubroff, P. M. (1983). The effects of a jogging program on psychiatric inpatients with symptoms of depression. *Occupational Therapy Journal of Research, 3,* 173-175.

Keywords: activity, affect, competence

This study found that the symptoms of depression were lessened during participation in a jogging program. The authors suggest that the sense of mastery acquired through regular jogging has a broad impact on daily life.

187. Kielhofner, G., & Nelson, C. (1983). A study of patient motivation and cooperation/participation in occupational therapy. *Occupational Therapy Journal of Research, 3,* 35-46.

Keyword: motivation

This article explores the relationship between the value placed on occupational therapy, and cooperation and participation exhibited during treatment.

188. Salz, C. (1983). A theoretical approach to the treatment of work difficulties in borderline personality disorder. *Occupational Therapy in Mental Health, 3,* 33-46.

Keywords: psychodynamic, work

This paper develops a psychodynamic perspective on the work difficulties associated with borderline personality disorder and proposes high levels of exploratory behaviour as a primary occupational dysfunction for this population.

189. Van Deusen-Fox, J. (1983). Selected measures of patient motivation and creativity and their relationship to occupational therapy outcome. *Occupational Therapy Journal of Research, 3,* 121-122.

Keywords: activity, motivation

The results of this study suggest that internal locus of control and voluntary participation predict better treatment outcomes in occupational therapy.

190. Burton, J. E. (1984). Occupational therapy in long term psychiatry: What's new? *Canadian Journal of Occupational Therapy, 51,* 176-179.

Keywords: behaviour, values

The results of a survey found that the clinical role of occupational therapists focused on affecting behavioural and attitudinal changes in clients.

191. Henry, A. D., Nelson, D. L., & Duncombe, L. W. (1984). Choice making in group and individual activity. *Am J Occup Ther, 38,* 245-251.

Keywords: empowerment, group, self

The results of this study suggest that individual sense of power decreased in response to freedom of choice being removed during group activities. It is proposed that that the group context heightened individual self-awareness.

192. Kremer, E. R., Nelson, D. L., & Duncombe, L. W. (1984). Effects of selected activities on affective meaning in psychiatric patients. *Am J Occup Ther, 38,* 522-528.

Keywords: activity, affect, meaning

This study examined the affective responses elicited by participation in common occupational therapy activities used with people with psychiatric disorders.

193. Kirchner, M. A. (1984). Motivation as a factor of perceived exertion in purposeful versus non-purposeful activity. *Am J Occup Ther, 38,* 165-170.

Keywords: activity, motivation, work

This study provided evidence for the assumption that intrinsic motivation, expressed as participation in purposeful activity, positively influences perceived exertion to enhance performance.

194. Silva, J. M., & Klatsky, J. (1984). Body image and physical activity. *Physical and Occupational Therapy in Pediatrics, 4,* 85-92.

Keywords: activity, self

This article explores the concept of body image, the factors that influence body image, and the potential for physical activity to enhance body image.

195. Adelstein, L. A., & Nelson, D. L. (1985). Effects of sharing versus non-sharing on affective meaning in collage activities. *Occupational Therapy in Mental Health, 5,* 29-45.

Keywords: activity, affect, meaning

This study found no differences in the affective dimensions (power, action, and meaning) of a group collage activity under sharing and nonsharing conditions.

196. Blakeney, A. B. (1985). Adolescent development: An application of the model of human occupation. *Occupational Therapy in Health Care, 2,* 19-40.

Keywords: adolescent, competence, self

In this article, adolescence is discussed from the perspective of the psychoemotional factors of need for exploration and mastery, development of values and interest, occupational choice, and internalization of roles.

197. Barris, R. (1986). Occupational dysfunction and eating disorders: Theory and approach to treatment. *Occupational Therapy in Mental Health, 6,* 27-45.

Keywords: activity, competence, psychological

In this exploration of eating disorders using the framework of the model of human occupation, the author develops inconsistencies in the relationship between activity and mastery.

198. Froehlich, J., & Nelson, D. (1986). Affective meanings of life review through activities and discussion. *Am J Occup Ther, 40,* 27-33.

Keywords: activity, affect, meaning

This study compared affective meanings of life review through activities and through discussion on self-ratings.

199. Krupa, T., & Thornton, J. (1986). The Pleasure deficit in schizophrenia. *Occupational Therapy in Mental Health, 6,* 65-77.

     Keyword: affect

     The authors explore anhedonia, the loss of pleasure experienced by persons diagnosed with schizophrenia, its relationship to occupation, and potential occupational therapy interventions.

200. Magill, J., & Hurlbut, N. (1986). The self-esteem of adolescents with cerebral palsy. *Am J Occup Ther, 40,* 402-407.

     Keywords: adolescent, self, values

     This study suggested that the lower self-esteem of adolescent girls with cerebral palsy might be understood from the perspective of self-perceptions and the personal values placed on attractiveness.

201. Mosey, A. C. (1986). *Psychosocial components of occupational therapy.* New York: Raven Press.

     Keywords: learning, psychological

     In her overview of the psychosocial components of occupational therapy, Mosey includes a discussion of psychological functions and occupational performance. Mosey includes analytic frames of reference and links theory to the change process. She also includes a review of learning theories as they apply to the teaching-learning process in occupational therapy.

202. Ray, R. (1986). Older adult happiness: Contributions of activity breadth and intensity. *Physical and Occupational Therapy in Geriatrics, 4,* 31-43.

     Keywords: affect, aging, motivation

     This study examined the relationship between happiness and the intensity of commitment to activities in the older adult.

203. Riopel Smith, N., Kielhofner, G., & Hawkins Watts, J. (1986). The relationship between volition, activity pattern, and life satisfaction in the elderly. *Am J Occup Ther, 40,* 278-283.

     Keywords: activity, aging, volition

     This study provides evidence that interests, values, and personal causation reflected in daily occupations is related to positive life satisfaction.

204. Rowenbusch, D. (1986). Psychic energy—The activator of the low energy patient. *Occupational Therapy in Health Care, 3,* 55-63.

    Keyword: motivation

    This article examines the theoretical basis of psychic energy as a potential enabler of physical performance.

205. Sharrott, G. W. (1986). An analysis of occupational therapy theoretical approaches for mental health: Are the profession's major treatment approaches truly occupational therapy? *Occupational Therapy in Mental Health, 5*(4), 1-15.

    Keywords: emotion, models, psychological

    The article discusses prevalent theoretical approaches used in occupational therapy mental health settings, including several that are based on psychoemotional theory. The relationship of each of the approaches to occupational therapy perspectives is examined.

206. Sharrott, G. W., & Cooper-Fraps, C. (1986). Theories of motivation in occupational therapy: An overview. *Am J Occup Ther, 40*(4), 249-257.

    Keywords: models, motivation

    This article explores the motivational theories of five occupational therapy approaches: the occupational behaviour approach, object relations, action consequence, recapitulation of ontogenesis, and developmental facilitation.

207. Steinbeck, T. (1986). Purposeful activity and performance. *Am J Occup Ther, 40,* 529-534.

    Keywords: activity, motivation

    This study provides support for the assumption that purposeful activity enhances motivation to enable performance.

208. Bruce, M. A., & Borg, B. (1993). *Psychosocial occupational therapy: Frames of reference for intervention* (2nd ed.). Thorofare, NJ: SLACK Incorporated.

    Keywords: behavioural, cognitive-behavioural, psychodynamic

    Bruce and Borg provide and overview of several occupational therapy frames of reference that are consistent with psychoemotional therapy. They emphasize the need for occupational therapists to be well versed in multiple theories in order to provide humanistic and individualized treatment that is validated through research. This book includes chapters on the following frames of reference: object relations, behavioural, and cognitive behavioural.

209. Barris, R. (1987). Relationships between eating behaviours and person/environment interactions in college women. *Occupational Therapy Journal of Research, 7,* 273-288.

Keywords: emotion, environment, psychological

In this study, individuals with eating disorders were found to derive less joy, fulfilment, expectation of success, and control while engaged in personal projects.

210. Rocker, D. J., & Nelson, D. (1987). Affective responses to keeping and not keeping an activity product. *Am J Occup Ther, 41,* 152-157.

Keywords: activity, affect

The results of this study suggested a relationship between hostile feelings and increased energy, and the experience of not keeping the product of a personal project.

211. Johnston, M. T. (1987). Occupational therapists and the teaching of cognitive behavioural skills. *Occupational Therapy in Mental Health, 7,* 69-81.

Keywords: cognitive-behavioural

This article discusses cognitive-behavioural theory and suggestions for its application in occupational therapy practice.

212. Stowell, M. (1987). Psychosocial role of the occupational therapist with pediatric bone marrow transplant. *Occupational Therapy in Mental Health, 7,* 39-50.

Keyword: psychological

This article reviews psychological factors associated with childhood cancer and discusses occupational therapy interventions.

213. Doble, S. (1988). Intrinsic motivation and clinical practice: The key to understanding the unmotivated client. *Canadian Journal of Occupational Therapy, 55,* 75-80.

Keywords: activity, competence, motivation

This article presents a conceptual model of the process through which involvement in intrinsically motivating activities leads to a sense of competence.

214. Moyers, P. A. (1988). An organizational framework for occupational therapy in the treatment of alcoholism. *Occupational Therapy in Mental Health, 8,* 27-45.

Keywords: psychodynamic, psychological

This article presents alcoholism from a psychodynamic perspective and suggests occupational therapy interventions.

215. Nickel, I. (1988). Adapting structured learning therapy for use in a psychiatric adult day hospital. *Canadian Journal of Occupational Therapy, 55*, 21-25.

Keywords: adult, learning

In this article, the development and rationale of a structured learning therapy approach in a psychiatric day hospital program are presented.

216. Duncombe, L. W., Howe, M. C., & Schwartzberg, S. L. (1988). *Case Simulations in Psychosocial Occupational Therapy* (2nd ed.). Philadelphia: F. A. Davis.

Keywords: psychological, emotion, behaviour

This book provides overviews of psychoanalytic and behavioural theories as they are applied to occupational therapy practice.

217. Foy, S. (1990). Factors contributing to learned helplessness in the institutionalized aged: A review of the literature. *Physical and Occupational Thearpy in Geriatrics, 9*, 1-23.

Keywords: aging, personal causation, psychological

In this article, Foy reviews the literature related to the theory and experience of learned helplessness as it relates to the institutionalized aged.

218. Maynard, M. (1990). Exploring adult day care participants' responses to psychosocial stress. *Occupational Therapy in Mental Health, 10*, 65-84.

Keywords: aging, stress

This study examined the stress levels of the frail elderly and the extent to which participation in stress management procedures influenced stress levels.

219. Christiansen, C. (1991). Performance deficits as sources of stress: Coping theory and occupational therapy. In C. Christiansen & C. Baum (Eds.), *Occupational therapy: Overcoming human performance deficits* (pp. 69-100). Thorofare, NJ: SLACK Incorporated.

Keywords: adaptation, coping

This chapter examines the dynamics of coping with a view of preparing occupational therapists to enable successful adaptation in response to performance deficits.

220. Coster, W. (1991). Current concepts of children's perception of control. *Am J Occup Ther, 45,* 19-25.

Keywords: children, personal causation, self

This paper reviews theory, research, and assessment methods related to children's perceived control and personal efficacy.

221. Depoy, E., & Kolodner, E. (1991). Psychological performance factors. In C. Christiensen & C. Baum (Eds.), *Occupational therapy: Overcoming human performance deficits* (pp. 304-332). Thorofare, NJ: SLACK Incorporated.

Keywords: emotion, models, psychological

The cited chapter briefly reviews major psychoemotional theories and discusses the effects of psychological and emotional factors on occupational performance.

222. Fine, S. B. (1991). Eleanor Clarke Slagle lecture. Resilience and human adaptability: Who rises above adversity? *Am J Occup Ther, 45,* 493-450.

Keywords: coping, meaning, self, stress

Fine discusses the influence of perceptions of self and affect on resilience in the face of major life stress.

223. Magill-Evans, J. (1991). Self-esteem of persons with cerebral palsy: From adolescence to adulthood. *Am J Occup Ther, 45,* 819-825.

Keywords: adolescent, self

This longitudinal study examined self-esteem changes from adolescence to adulthood for people with cerebral palsy and explored the factors that lead to changes in self-esteem.

224. Brown, T. (1992). Assertiveness training for clients with a psychiatric illness: A pilot study. *British Journal of Occupational Therapy, 55,* 137-140.

Keywords: cognitive behavioural, learning, self

Brown presents the assertiveness and self-esteem outcomes for people with psychiatric illnesses following a 7-week assertiveness training program that was based on the model of human occupation and social learning theory.

225. Cara, E. (1992). Neutralizing the narcissistic style: Narcissistic personality disorder. *Occupational Therapy in Health Care, 8*, 135-156.

Keyword: psychological

The author discusses occupational therapy treatment for narcissistic personality disorder within the context of current psychological theory.

226. Dickerson, A. (1992). The relationship between affect and cognition. *Occupational Therapy in Mental Health, 12*, 47-59.

Keywords: affect, cognition, models

Dickerson reviews theories about affective-cognitive interaction and their implications for occupational therapy in mental health.

227. Froehlich, J. (1992). OT interventions with survivors of sexual abuse. *Occupational Therapy in Health Care, 8*, 1-25.

Keywords: emotion, psychodynamic

This paper applies the model of human occupation to address daily living concerns and object relations theory to address recall and emotional recovery.

228. Gage, M. (1992). The appraisal model of coping: An assessment and treatment model for occupational therapy. *Am J Occup Ther, 46*(4), 353-362.

Keyword: coping

The author presents a model of coping to assist therapists with understanding and intervening when coping problems interfere with occupational performance.

229. Janelle, S. (1992). Locus of control in nondisabled versus congenitally physically disabled adolescents. *Am J Occup Ther, 46*, 334-342.

Keywords: adolescent, disability, personal causation

This study examined the relationship between disability and locus of control in adolescents, and considered characteristics of individuals who have an internal locus of control.

230. Barnitt, R., & Mayers, C. (1993). Can occupational therapists be both humanists and Christians? A study of two conflicting frames. *British Journal of Occupational Therapy, 56*, 84-88.

Keywords: development, humanism, models, psychodynamic

The authors advance theory by discussing elements of humanism that may conflict with behavioural, developmental, and psychodynamic approaches.

---

231. Bonder, B. R. (1993). Issues in assessment of psychosocial components of function. *Am J Occup Ther, 47,* 211-216.

Keyword: psychological

The author discusses the lack of clarity in the definition and measurement of psychosocial variables and in their application to occupation.

---

232. King, G. (1993). Self-evaluation and self-concept of adolescents with physical disabilities. *Am J Occup Ther, 47,* 132-140.

Keywords: adolescent, disability, self

This study focuses on the relationship between several aspects of self-concept and physical disability and examines the relationship between social self-efficacy and independence and persistence in adolescence.

---

233. Miller, R. J., & Walker, K. F. (Eds.). (1993). *Perspectives on theory for the practice of occupational therapy.* Gaithersburg, MD: Aspen.

Keywords: emotion, models, psychological

This book includes reviews of the work of three occupational therapists: Gail Fidler, Anne Cronin Mosey, and Gary Kielhofner, who integrated psychoemotional constructs into their own theories related to occupation.

---

234. Saint-Jean, M., & Desrosiers, L. (1993). Psychoanalytic considerations regarding the occupational therapy setting for treatment of the psychotic patient. *Occupational Therapy in Mental Health, 45,* 438-449.

Keyword: psychodynamic

This paper applies principles of psychoanalysis to the occupational therapy treatment of persons with psychosis.

---

235. Gage, M., Noh, S., Polatajko, H., & Kaspar, V. (1994). Measuring perceived self-efficacy in occupational therapy. *Am J Occup Ther, 48,* 783-790.

Keywords: competence, self

This article contributes to the understanding of perceived self-efficacy by presenting the development of a measure of self-efficacy and its psychometric properties.

236. Gage, M., & Polatajko, H. (1994). Enhancing occupational performance through an understanding of perceived self-efficacy. *Am J Occup Ther, 48,* 452-461.

   Keywords: competence, self
   This article discusses the construct of self-efficacy and its relationship to occupational therapy.

237. Helfrich, C., Kielhofner, G., & Mattingly, C. (1994), Volition as narrative: Understanding motivation in chronic illness. *Am J Occup Ther, 48,* 311-317.

   Keywords: motivation, volition
   The authors expand the concept of volition through the investigation of the life histories of two persons with psychiatric disorders.

238. Moss-Morris, R., & Petrie, K. (1994). Illness perceptions: Implications for occupational therapy. *Australian Occupational Therapy Journal, 41,* 73-82.

   Keywords: coping, emotion
   The authors consider how illness perception influences coping, emotional states, and health outcomes. Ideas are advanced about how these perceptions could be used in OT practice.

239. Wright, S. (1994). Physical and emotional abuse and neglect of preschool children: A literature review. *Australian Occupational Therapy Journal, 41,* 55-63.

   Keywords: emotion, psychological
   Wright reviews the literature to examine the affects of maltreatment on preschool children in several areas including emotional development.

240. Benetton, M. (1995). A case study applying a psychodynamic approach to occupational therapy. *Occupational Therapy International, 2,* 220-228.

   Keyword: psychodynamic
   This article presents aspects of psychoemotional theory through a case study.

241. Dickerson, A. (1995). Action identification may explain why the doing of activities in occupational therapy effects positive change in clients. *British Journal of Occupational Therapy, 58,* 461-464.

Keywords: activity, meaning, self

This paper presents a psychological theory that relates the nature of the action in activity to levels of identity. The author suggests applications of this action theory to occupational therapy theory and practice.

---

242. Dutton, R. (1995). **Psychosocial issues. In R. Dutton (Ed.),** *Clinical reasoning in physical disabilities* **(pp. 209-219). Baltimore: Williams & Wilkins.**

Keywords: disability, stress, volition

Dutton argues the importance of considering psychosocial issues in practice in the area of physical disabilities. Psychoemotional factors considered include volition, sexuality, and stress response.

---

243. Jackson, J. (1995). **Sexual orientation: Its relevance to occupational science and the practice of occupational therapy.** *Am J Occup Ther,* **49, 669-679.**

Keywords: meaning, self, sexuality

Jackson examines the relevance of sexual orientation to occupation and suggests that it may be understood as an aspect of meaning that is expressed through occupation.

---

244. Rebeiro, K. L. (1995). **Occupation as means to mental health: A review of the literature and a call for research.** *Canadian Journal of Occupational Therapy,* **65, 12-19.**

Keywords: meaning, self

This article examines the extent to which the assumption that occupation promotes mental health through the realization of meaning, purpose, and self-actualization has been developed in the occupational therapy literature.

---

245. Telford, R., & Ainscough, K. (1995). **Non-directive play therapy and psychodynamic theory: Never the twain shall meet?** *British Journal of Occupational Therapy,* **58, 201-203.**

Keywords: children, play, psychodynamic

The authors suggest that analytical theory be combined with nondirective play therapy to enhance the theoretical foundation of play therapy in occupational therapy within child psychiatry.

---

246. Trombly, C. A. (1995). **Eleanor Clarke Slagle lecture. Purposefulness and meaningfulness as therapeutic mechanisms.** *Am*

J Occup Ther, 49, 960-972.

Keywords: meaning, motivation

In this article, occupation is discussed as a means to enhance motivation by providing purpose and meaning.

---

247. Cronin, A. F. (1996). Psychosocial and emotional domains of behaviour. In J. Case-Smith, A. S. Allen, & P. N. Pratt (Eds.), *Occupational therapy for children* (3rd ed., pp. 387-429.). St. Louis, MO: C. V. Mosby.

Keywords: children, development, models

This book chapter reviews psychological and emotional factors in child development. It includes a review of theoretical approaches and corresponding OT interventions including behavioural and learning theory and psychodynamic theory.

---

248. Early, M. B. (1996). *Mental health concepts and techniques for the occupational therapy assistant* (2nd ed.). Philadelphia: Lippincott Raven.

Keywords: behavioural, psychodynamic

This book provides a brief review of object relations and behavioural theories, and how they relate to mental health and illness.

---

249. Mostert E., Zacharkiewicz, A., & Fossey, E. (1996). Claiming the illness experience: Using narrative to enhance theoretical understanding. *Australian Occupational Therapy Journal, 43*, 125-132.

Keyword: phenomenology

The article discusses how health practitioners can affect clients' perceptions of illness to influence health-related outcomes.

---

250. Polkinghorne, D. (1996). Transformative narratives: From victimic to agentic life plots. *Am J Occup Ther, 50*, 299-305.

Keywords: competence, personal causation, phenomenology

The author explores the use of narratives to move individuals with occupational dysfunction from a passive and acquiescent stance toward their lives to one of active agency and self-determination.

---

251. Price-Lackey, P., & Cashman, J. (1996). Jenny's story: Reinventing oneself through occupational and narrative configuration. *Am J Occup Ther, 50*, 306-314.

Keywords: identity, phenomenology, self

This article presents two life history interviews that revealed the processes of identity reconstruction through occupation for a woman who experienced a traumatic head injury.

252. Salo-Chydenius, S. (1996). Changing helplessness to coping: An exploratory study of social skills training with individuals with long-term mental illness. *Occupational Therapy International, 3,* 174-189.

Keywords: cognitive-behavioural, coping

The focus of this study was the application of social skills training based on a cognitive-behavioural frame of reference to enable individuals with long-term mental illness to generalize communication skills to everyday life.

253. Schwammle, D. (1996). Occupational competence explored. *Canadian Journal of Occupational Therapy, 63,* 323-330.

Keywords: competence, motivation

The author reviews the theory of competence motivation and relates it to occupational models of competence and enablement.

254. Bonder, B. R. (1997). Coping with psychological and emotional challenges. In C. Christiansen & C. Baum (Eds.), *Occupational therapy: Enabling function and well-being* (2nd ed., pp. 312-335). Thorofare, NJ: SLACK Incorporated.

Keywords: emotion, models, psychological

This book chapter reviews three psychological theories and five occupational theory conceptual models with respect to their views on key psychological constructs, function, and dysfunction.

255. Alessandri, M., & Skinner, J. T. (1998). Psychological models. In E. Cara & A. MacRae (Eds.), *Psychosocial occupational therapy* (pp. 59-96). Albany, NY: Delmar.

Keywords: psychological, emotion, behaviour, cognitive-behavioural

This book chapter provides a brief review of psychoemotional theories relevant to the practice of psychosocial occupational therapy.

256. Emerson, H., Cook, J, Polatajko, H., & Segal, R. (1998). Enjoyment experiences as described by persons with schizophrenia: A qualitative study. *Canadian Journal of Occupational Therapy, 65,*

183-192.

Keywords: affect, psychological

Using the concept of *flow* as a theoretical framework, this study explored enjoyment as experienced by persons with schizophrenia.

257. Neistadt, M. E., & Crepeau, E. B. (1998). *Willard & Spackman's occupational therapy* (9th ed.). Philadelphia: Lippincott Williams & Wilkins.

Keywords: behaviour, learning, models, psychological

This text offers several chapters related to psychoemotional theory including behavioural learning theories and occupational therapy interventions focused on the psychosocial components of mental health, pain, and stress.

258. Henderson, S. (1999). Frames of reference utilized in the rehabilitation of individuals with eating disorders. *Canadian Journal of Occupational Therapy, 66*, 43-51.

Keywords: models, psychological

The author reviews the prevalent psychological theories applied in the understanding and treatment of eating disorders.

259. Lloyd, C., & Papas, V. (1999). Art as therapy within occupational therapy in mental health settings: A review of the literature. *British Journal of Occupational Therapy, 62*, 31-35.

Keywords: activity, emotion, meaning

This article discusses art as a meaningful activity that promotes emotional expression.

260. Murphy, S., Trombly, C., Tickle-Degnen, L., & Jacobs, K. (1999). The effect of keeping an end-product on intrinsic motivation. *Am J Occup Ther, 53*, 153-158.

Keywords: activity, motivation

The researchers examine the relationship of keeping the end-product of an activity on intrinsic motivation and other psychological factors.

261. Saunders, I., Sayer, M., & Goodale, A. (1999). The relationship between playfulness and coping in preschool children: A pilot study. *Am J Occup Ther, 53*, 221-226.

Keywords: children, coping, play

This study examines playfulness as an indicator of coping in young children.

262. Eklund, M. (2000). Applying object relations theory to psychosocial occupational therapy: Empirical and theoretical considerations. *Occupational Therapy in Mental Health, 15,* 1-26.

Keywords: psychodynamic, models
Eklund considers the merits of including object relations theory as an occupational therapy conceptual model.

263. Chin-yu, W., Shu-Ping, C., & Grossman, J. (2000). Facilitating intrinsic motivation in clients with mental illness. *Occupational Therapy in Mental Health, 16,* 1-14.

Keywords: models, motivation
This paper develops the motivational problems experienced by people with mental illness from the perspective of self-determination theory and learned helplessness theory.

264 Christiansen, C. (2000). Identity, personal projects and happiness: Self-construction in everyday action. *Journal of Occupational Science, 7*(3), 98-107.

Keywords: activity, affect, identity
This study examines the identity-related dimensions of personal projects, the influence of self-identity on subjective well-being, and the age-related patterns of identity dimensions predicting subjective well-being.

265. Spalding, N. (2000). The empowerment of clients through preoperative education. *British Journal of Occupational Therapy, 63,* 148-154.

Keyword: empowerment
This article reports on a study of the strategies used to increase personal empowerment within a preoperative educational program for people awaiting hip replacement surgery.

266. Williamson, P. (2000). Football and tin cans: A model of identity formation based on sexual orientation and expressed through engagement in occupations. *British Journal of Occupational Therapy, 63,* 432-438.

Keywords: identity, self, sexuality

This paper presents the importance of occupations within the context of a 6-stage model of identity formation based on sexual orientation.

---

267. Willoughby, C., Polatajko, H., Currado, C., Harris, K., & King, G. (2000). Measuring the self-esteem of adolescents with mental health problems: Theory meets practice. *Canadian Journal of Occupational Therapy, 67,* 230-238.

Keywords: adolescents, self

This study questions the assumption that adolescents with mental health problems have low self-esteem and addresses the relationship of self-concept to self-esteem.

SOME IMPORTANT IDEAS ABOUT THE PSYCHOLOGICAL-EMOTIONAL DETERMINANTS OF OCCUPATION:

- This area of theory locates the source of occupational performance problems in the person.
- In particular, this area of theory focuses on thoughts and feelings, and their effects on occupation.
- This theory area addresses the topic of motivation and personal causation, including basic ideas about why humans engage in occupation.
- While issues of mental illness are a part of this theory area, its relevance is broader —pertaining to any instance where thoughts or feelings affect occupation.
- It is important to distinguish between thought patterns and cognitive dysfunction. The former is psychological-emotional construct, the latter is a cognitive-neurological one.
- Occupational conceptual models help us to understand how concepts like identity, motivation, coping, and beliefs about personal causation affect what we do.
- Basic conceptual models tell us about three main areas of human psychological and emotional functioning: thoughts (cognitive approach), feelings (psychodynamic approach), and behaviour (behavioural approach).
- Each of these has a counterpart in occupational therapy theory: cognitive-behavioural approach, object-relations, and acquisitional approach.
- The occupational model of practice includes activity analysis and some particular projective techniques.

HERE IS A PRACTICAL PROBLEM THAT MAY HELP TO RAISE SOME OF THE
IMPORTANT IDEAS IN THE AREA OF PSYCHOLOGICAL-EMOTIONAL
DETERMINANTS OF OCCUPATION:

Neville is a lecturer in the psychology department at XYZ University. He completed his PhD in psychology several years ago; and for the past 2 years, he has taught Introductory Psychology to undergraduate students in the health sciences. Starting this September, Neville will also be teaching the occupational therapy students their courses on psychological theory, psychiatry and mental health, and applications in occupational therapy. In preparation, Neville spends the summer reading up on occupational therapy in mental health. The students he teaches will have already had Introductory Psychology, as well as a half course in psychiatry. His task, therefore, is to identify the knowledge needed by occupational therapy students in the mental health area. He knows from his reading that there are a number of different approaches to occupational therapy with clients with mental illness and that these are often related to the major psychological theories with which he is already familiar. He is surprised by how little he finds in the literature on feelings and emotions. He is aware that coping, adjustment, and motivation are important concepts for occupational therapists. He also discovers a concept that is new to him—activity analysis.

THE COGNITIVE-NEUROLOGICAL DETERMINANTS OF OCCUPATION

| 11 |

Lorna Doubt, MSc

Introduction

In this theory area, occupation is analyzed from the perspective of the cognitive, perceptual, and neurological skills that contribute to successful occupational performance. It is assumed that perceptual, cognitive, motor control, and sensory integration problems result in impairment of function of the central nervous system. Ideas that link the ability of the individual to perform meaningful activities to their skills in interpreting, processing, integrating, and applying sensory information would be included in this category. Theoretical work that explores and explains the relationship of concepts of motor control and motor learning to occupation would also be classified under this heading. Literature focusing on the association between occupation and cognitive phenomena such as attention, memory, initiation, planning, reflection and adaptive problem solving, organizing, and assimilating information that enables one to think and act can be found in this section. The cognitive-neurological theory area includes research findings and propositions that reflect the relationship of occupation to perception, including concepts such as tactile sensitivity, proprioception, vestibular and visual perception, praxis, and body scheme.

A Brief History of Theory of Cognitive-Neurological Theory

Literature in this theoretical area is notably sparse prior to the 1950s. Although articles referring to specific neurological diagnoses such as *spastic hand* (Johnson, 1937), *hemiplegic arm* (Covalt, Yamshon, Nowicki, 1949), and *cerebral palsy* (Marin, 1940) emerged in the 1940s, the predominant focus on vocational activities and mental health prevailed. However, with the increased prevalence of physical disability and chronic conditions after World War II, occupational therapy practice began to reflect the increasing interest in physical function and treatment techniques.

The developments in neurological basic science research in the 1950s and 1960s enabled occupational therapists to understand more clearly the cause of dysfunction in their patients with neurological and cognitive deficits. Medical science knowledge and techniques for diagnosis and treatment of acute illness developed rapidly during these decades, and the occupational therapy profession responded with an increasing focus on science and acute illness in education, practice, and research. In keeping with the biomedical, reductionist approach favoured by medical science, the occupational therapy literature of this era emphasized therapy techniques to change performance components, rather than a holistic approach to understanding occupation. In fact, this was a period of conflict and professional insecurity for occupational therapists about the "complexity of illness relative to the simplicity of our tools" (Reilly, 1962).

During these decades, there is evidence of a dramatic increase in writings related to neurological, sensory motor, and cognitive-perceptual function. Publications by authors, such as Ayres (1954, 1956, 1961), Brunnstrom (1961), Llorens et al. (1964), and Rood (1956) tended to focus on neurophysiological explanations and strategies for assessment and intervention to improve motor performance. Little theory was developed to explain the relationship between occupation and neurological or cognitive function.

The 1970s and 1980s were a period of dramatic theoretical growth for occupational therapy in many areas. Information resulting from the rapid expansion of knowledge in the neurosciences and understanding of the neuromuscular system became increasingly available to occupational therapists. However, the biomedical model, characterized by technological discoveries, quantifiable measurement, and acute medical care, continued to dominate in the health disciplines, making it difficult to rationalize occupation-based therapies. Occupational therapy practitioners were left to bridge the gap between the new neurological theories and occupation, and the literature persisted in focusing on treatment and components of occupation rather than occupation.

The late 1980s brought a shift to community practice and promoted a change in thinking and role definition for occupational therapists. The literature began to reflect an increasing interest in developing ideas about occupation. Articles encouraging the integration of occupational therapy knowledge and neurobehavioral sciences, and exploring the role of theory in neurobehavioral treatment approaches, became more prevalent. By the 1990s, a growing body of research literature aimed at understanding the relationship between neurological and cognitive deficits and occupational performance problems became available to students and practitioners.

References

Ayres, A. J. (1954). Ontogenetic principles in the development of arm and hand function. *Am J Occup Ther*, 8, 95-9.

Ayres, A. J. (1955). Proprioceptive facilitation elicited through the upper extremities: Parts 1, 2 & 3. *Am J Occup Ther*, 9, 1-9, 57-8, 121-6

Ayres, A. J. (1961). Development of body scheme in children. *Am J Occup Ther*, 15, 99-102.

Brunnstrom, S. (1961). Motor behavior in adult hemiplegic patients, hints for training. *Am J Occup Ther*, 14, 6-10.

Covalt, D. A., Yamshon, L. J., & Nowicki, V. (1949). Physiological aid to the functional training of the hemiplegic arm. *Am J Occup Ther*, 3, 286-8.

Johnson, G. V. (1937). Occupational therapy for the spastic hand. *Occupational Therapy & Rehabilitation*, 16, 1-13.

Llorens, L., Rubin, E., Braun, J., Beck, G., Mottley, N., & Beall, D. (1964). Cognitive perceptual motor functions: A preliminary report on training. *Am J Occup Ther, 18*, 202-7.

Marin, E. F. (1940). Occupational therapy treatment for cerebral palsy at the Children's Rehabilitation Institute. *Occupational Therapy & Rehabilitation, 19*, 331-8.

Reilly, M. (1962). Occupational therapy can be one of the great ideas of 20th century medicine. *Am J Occup Ther, 16*, 1-9.

Rood, M. (1956). Neurophysiological mechanisms utilized in the treatment of neuromuscular dysfunction. *Am J Occup Ther, 10*, 220-4.

KEYWORDS USED IN THIS CHAPTER

Activity	Family	Motor	Self-care
Apraxia	Habit	Neuroscience	Sensory
Behavioural	Handwriting	Neurodevelopmental	Sensory integration
Children	Hemiplegia	Perception	Social
Cognitive	Independence	Play	Work
Coordination	Learning	Rehabilitation	
Environment	Models	Self	

Bibliographic Entries for the Cognitive-Neurological Determinants of Occupation

268. Carlsen, P. N. (1975). Comparison of two occupational therapy approaches for treating the young cerebral-palsied child. *Am J Occup Ther, 29*, 267-272.

Keyword: children

This article reports on a pilot study to determine whether the facilitation or the functional occupational therapy treatment approach is more effective for children with cerebral palsy. Ten pairs of children with similar developmental ages were randomly assigned to two treatment programs. The findings indicated that those children who received facilitation treatment showed greater improvement in developmental skills than those in the functional treatment group.

269. Baum, C. (1981). Relationship between constructional praxis and dressing in head-injured patients. *Am J Occup Ther, 35*(7), 438-442.

Keywords: perception, self-care

The study described in this article explored the potential relationship between dressing ability and constructional praxis performance in the head-injured population. The findings indicate that perceptual deficits in people with severe head injuries contribute to their inability to dress.

270. Scardina, V. (1981). From pegboards to integration. *Am J Occup Ther, 35,* 581-588.

Keywords: perception, sensory integration

A discussion of the nature of visual perception and the theory of sensory integration as it relates to occupational therapy is followed by a description of current occupational therapy treatment strategies for sensory integrative disorders. The article emphasizes the importance of integrating occupational therapy knowledge and practice into the neurobehavioural sciences.

271. Allen, C. K. (1982). Independence through activity: The practice of occupational therapy. *Am J Occup Ther, 36,* 731-739.

Keywords: activity, cognition, independence

The author presents an outline for an emerging theory to guide occupational therapy practice with mental disorders. The hierarchy of cognitive levels with an accompanying task analysis describes functional distinctions in the severity of disorder, as reflected in routine task behaviour.

272. DiJoseph, L. M. (1982). Independence through activity: Mind, body, and environment interaction in therapy. *Am J Occup Ther, 36,* 740-744.

Keywords: activity, environment, independence, motor

The relationship of philosophy, theory, and practice is explained. The author argues that purposeful activity, the primary occupational therapy tool, must be integrated into concepts of motor behaviour.

273. Kaplan, K. (1982). Visuospatial deficits after right hemisphere stroke. *Am J Occup Ther, 36(5),* 314-321.

Keywords: perception, hemiplegia

In this study of the impact of visuospatial deficits on functional status following right hemisphere stroke, little correlation between severity of hemiparesis and severity of visuospatial deficits was found. However, the results suggest that both motor and visuospatial dysfunction are important factors influencing functional outcomes.

274. Mack, W., Lindquist, J. E., & Parham, L. D. (1982). A synthesis of occupational behavior and sensory integration concepts in theory and practice. Part 1: Theoretical foundation. *Am J Occup Ther, 36,* 365-374.

275. Lindquist, J. E., Mack, W., & Parham, L. D. (1982). A synthesis of occupational behaviors and sensory integration concepts in theory and practice. Part 2: Clinical applications. *Am J Occup Ther, 36,* 433-437.

Keywords: children, play, sensory integration

These two articles describe a model of play development for occupational therapy with disabled children based on sensory integration and occupational behaviour theories. The authors review and compare the major concepts of sensory integration and occupational behaviour, and present a model of play development using general systems theory as a framework.

276. Williamson, G. G. (1982). A heritage of activity: Development of theory. *Am J Occup Ther, 36,* 716-722.

Keywords: activity, models

This article examines ideas about the role of theory as the foundation of a profession. The author suggests that neurobehavioural treatment approaches used in occupational therapy practice should reflect theory about activity and occupation.

277. Gliner, J. A. (1985). Purposeful activity in motor learning theory: An event approach to motor skills acquisition. *Am J Occup Ther, 39,* 28-34.

Keywords: activity, learning, motor

The ecological or event approach to motor skill learning is presented as a treatment method occupational therapists can use in the rehabilitation of physical dysfunction. Purposeful activity is viewed as a prerequisite for skilled movement. The event approach considers the actor and the environment inseparable in learning motor skills. Implications for occupational therapy practice are given through a case example. The author concludes that further research is required to understand why purposeful activity facilitates motor skill acquisition.

278. Llorens, L. (1986). Activity analysis: Agreement among factors in a sensory processing model. *Am J Occup Ther, 40,* 103-110.

Keywords: activity, sensory

This paper describes a model for the study of intersensory processing of stimuli presented by selected tasks, activities, and occupation components. The results of a study based on this model suggest that tasks, activities, and occupation components possess inherent factors that may be used by occupational therapists to affect the interrelationships between external actions, external objects, and internal mental operations.

279. Anderson, J., Hinojosa, J., & Strauch, C. (1987). Integrating play in neurodevelopmental treatment. *Am J Occup Ther, 41,* 421-426.

Keywords: activity, neurodevelopmental, play

The authors maintain that play interaction with children with cerebral palsy is compatible with the application of neurodevelopmental treatment (NDT) principles. Concepts of therapeutic use of activity and neurophysiological theory provide the basis for play intervention.

280. Abreu, B., & Toglia, J. (1987). Cognitive rehabilitation: A model for occupational therapy. *Am J Occup Ther, 41,* 439-448.

Keywords: cognition, perception, rehabilitation

A cognitive rehabilitation model based on information-processing theory and learning concepts is described as a foundation for occupational therapy practice with brain-damaged adults. Treatment strategies based on the evaluation of function and dysfunction in six critical areas, including occupational behaviour, are discussed. The model is compared to three other approaches used by occupational therapists working with clients with perceptual deficits.

281. Burke, J. P. (1988). Combining the model of human occupation with the cognitive disability theory. *Occupational Therapy in Mental Health, 8,* 6-9.

Keywords: activity, cognition, rehabilitation

The author compares the model of human occupation and cognitive disability theory and explores the idea of combining the two theories. The conclusion is reached that both theories contain valuable information about human behaviour and the role of activity in the rehabilitative process.

282. Bundy, A. C. (1989). Comparison of the play skills of normal boys with boys with sensory intergrative dysfunction. *Occupational Therapy Journal of Research, 9,* 84-100.

Keywords: children, play, sensory integration

This article explores the relationship of sensory integrative capabilities to play skills among 4-to-6-year-old boys. The study concluded that the children with sensory integrative disorders were significantly less able than the normal children to manage space, manage materials, and interact socially in play, partially due to gross and fine motor incoordination.

283. Clifford, J. M., & Bundy, A. C. (1989). Play preference and play performance in normal boys and boys with sensory integrative dysfunction. *Occupational Therapy Journal of Research, 9,* 202-217.

Keywords: children, play, sensory integration

The importance of play is underlined as a precursor to future occupational behaviour. A study of 4-, 5-, and 6-year-old boys concluded that play preference was similar among two groups of children with and without sensory integrative dysfunction. Children with sensory integrative dysfunction scored significantly lower on overall play skills, participation, and material and space management.

---

284. **Neistadt, M. E. (1990). A critical analysis of occupational therapy approaches for perceptual deficits in adults with brain injury.** *Am J Occup Ther, 44, 299-304.*

Keyword: perception

The underlying theoretical assumptions of various adaptive and remedial approaches to occupational therapy treatment for perceptual deficits are discussed. Several general research questions about neurological mechanisms underlying recovery, treatment activities, and the relationship between perception and function are suggested.

---

285. **Ziviani, J. (1990). Handwriting: A perceptual-motor disturbance in children with myelomeningocele.** *Occupational Therapy Journal of Research, 10(1), 12-26.*

Keywords: children, perception, handwriting

The purpose of the study described in this article was to explain the handwriting difficulties experienced by children with myelomeningocele. The variables related to writing ability are identified and skill acquisition process is discussed.

---

286. **Hamilton, A. (1991). Sensory hand function of the child with spina bifida myelomeningocele.** *British Journal of Occupational Therapy, 54(9), 346-349.*

Keywords: children, sensory, handwriting

The study described in this article concluded that there are significant differences in sensory function between children with spina bifida and those without. It is suggested that sensory impairment may be the most salient cause of hand dysfunction and clumsy hand use identified in previous research.

---

287. **Titus, M. (1991). Correlation of perceptual performance and ADL in stroke patients.** *Am J Occup Ther, 45(5), 410-418.*

Keywords: perception, self-care

This study used perceptual and ADL tests to investigate the relationship between perceptual function and the performance of activities of daily living in 25 post-stroke males. The results indicated that some perceptual deficits correlated with ADL performance.

288. Bonney, M-A. (1992). Understanding and assessing handwriting difficulty: Perspectives from the literature. *Australian Occupational Therapy Journal, 39*(3), 7-15.

    Keywords: perception, coordination, handwriting

    Critical to assessment and remediation of handwriting dysfunction is an understanding of the relationship between variables assessed (i.e., motor coordination, biomechanical factors, perceptual processing, and psychoemotional issues) and handwriting performance. A review of the literature related to handwriting performance, dysfunction, and assessment is presented.

289. DePoy, E., & Burke, J. (1992). Viewing cognition through the lens of the model of human occupation. In N. Katz (Ed.), *Cognitive rehabilitation: Models for intervention in occupational therapy* (pp. 240-257). Stoneham, MA: Butterworth-Heinemann.

    Keywords: cognitive, rehabilitation

    The authors briefly review two major conceptualizations of cognition—constructivist and information processing—and integrate both in a definition of cognition. The model of human occupation is explained and used as a framework for an analysis of cognition.

290. Burke, J. P. (1993). Play: The life role of the infant and young child. In J. Case-Smith (Ed.), *Pediatric occupational therapy and early intervention.* (pp. 198-224). Newton, MA: Butterworth-Heinemann.

    Keywords: motor, play

    This chapter deals with play as a developmental function in infants and children. It includes sections on the motor explanation for reasons that children play, and play among children with special needs.

291. Glass, R. P., & Wolf, L. S. (1993). Feeding and oral-motor skills. In J. Case-Smith (Ed.), *Pediatric occupational therapy and early intervention.* (pp. 225-288). Newton, MA: Butterworth-Heinemann.

    Keywords: motor, self-care

    This chapter relates oral-motor component skills to the occupation of feeding.

292. Galski, T., Bruno, R., & Ehle, H. (1993). Prediction of behind-the-wheel driving performance in patients with cerebral brain damage: A discriminant function analysis. *Am J Occup Ther, 47*(5), 391-396.

Keywords: cognition, behavioural

The aim of this study was to determine the effectiveness of the evaluation methods used to measure clients' fitness to resume driving after brain injury or stroke. The results demonstrated that behaviours as well as residual cognitive deficits should be considered in determining fitness to drive.

293. Miller, R. J., & Walker, K. F. (Eds.). (1993). *Perspectives on theory for the practice of occupational therapy.* Gaithersburg, MA: Aspen.

Keyword: models

This book features seven theorists who have made major contributions to occupational therapy theory. Chapters on A. Jean Ayres and Claudia Allen relate to the cognitive-neurological determinants of occupation.

294. Penso, D. (1993). *Perceptuo-motor difficulties: Theory and strategies to help children, adolescents, and adults.* London: Chapman & Hall.

Keywords: children, motor, perception

This book focuses on the occupational performance problems experienced by children and young adults who have perceptual-motor dysfunction. The author discusses the relationship of gross and fine motor and perceptual deficits to activities such as eating, dressing, school performance, and career options.

295. Coster, W., Haley, S., & Baryza, M. J. (1994). Functional performance of young children after traumatic brain injury: A 6-month follow-up study. *Am J Occup Ther, 48*(3), 211-218.

Keywords: cognition, family

Standardized measures of functional performance and family functioning (child behavior checklist, pediatric evaluation of disability inventory, and impact on family scale) were used to assess children with brain injuries and their families at 1 and 6 months post-discharge. The authors concluded that there is a need for early identification of at-risk children and support for families of children with changes in functional behavior.

296. Katz, N. (1994). Cognitive rehabilitation: Models for intervention and research on cognition in occupational therapy. *Occupational Therapy International, 1*(1), 49-63.

Keywords: cognition, perception, rehabilitation

This article presents current theory and research to explore the cognitive-perceptual components of occupational performance and support the integration of cognitive rehabilitation concepts into occupational therapy practice. Occupational therapy cognitive rehabilitation models of practice are reviewed in terms of functional and remedial approaches.

297. **Mathiowetz, V., & Haugen, J. (1994). Motor behavior research: Implications for therapeutic approaches to central nervous system dysfunction. *Am J Occup Ther*, 48(8), 733-745.**

Keywords: learning, motor, models

The models and theories of motor behavior that are fundamental to the traditional approaches to central nervous system dysfunction are reviewed, and their assumptions and limitations discussed. The authors present and compare a contemporary task-oriented approach based on the systems model.

298. **Tseng, M., & Murray, E. (1994). Differences in perceptual-motor measures in children with good and poor handwriting. *Occupational Therapy Journal of Research*, 14(1), 19-36.**

Keywords: perception, motor, handwriting

This paper describes a study to examine the relationship between perceptual-motor abilities and handwriting skills of 143 Chinese children in grades three to five. The poor handwriters scored lower on most of the perceptual-motor tests, with motor planning being the salient factor contributing to their writing legibility.

299. **Baum, C. (1995). The contribution of occupation to function in persons with Alzheimer's disease. *Journal of Occupational Science*, 2(2), 59-67.**

Keywords: behaviour, self-care

This study explored the relationship of memory, executive skills, and occupation in people with Alzheimer's disease-type dementia. Those who persisted in occupational activity demonstrated disturbing behaviours less frequently were more independent in self-care activities, and their caregivers reported less stress.

300. **Case-Smith, J. (1995). The relationship among sensorimotor components, fine motor skills, and functional performance in preschool children. *Am J Occup Ther*, 49(7), 645-652.**

Keywords: children, handwriting, motor, sensory

Sensorimotor and fine motor skills and functional performance were evaluated for 30 preschool children with motor delays. Although significant correlations were found among sensorimotor components and discrete fine motor skills, few correlations emerged between foundational components of fine motor skill and functional performance in self-care, mobility, and social function. Possible explanations for the findings are discussed.

301. Jarus, T., & Loiter, Y. (1995). The effect of kinesthetic stimulation on acquisition and retention of a gross motor skill. *Canadian Journal of Occupational Therapy, 62*(1), 23-29.

     Keywords: coordination, learning, motor

     The authors investigated the role of kinesthetic stimulation in motor learning and performance of the gross motor task of kicking a ball. The results indicated that kinesthetic stimulation enhanced task acquisition, and possible explanations were discussed.

302. Malloy-Miller, T., Polatajko, H., & Anstett, B. (1995). Handwriting error patterns of children with mild motor difficulties. *Canadian Journal of Occupational Therapy, 62*(5), 258-267.

     Keywords: children, handwriting, perception

     The purpose of the study described in this article was to examine the relationship between handwriting error patterns and perceptual-motor abilities in children ages 7 to 12 years. The results demonstrated a correlation between visual-motor, sensory discrimination, and fine motor skills, and two of the three handwriting error patterns identified.

303. Rubio, K., & VanDeusen, J. (1995). Relation of perceptual and body image dysfunction to activities of daily living of persons after stroke. *Am J Occup Ther, 49*(6), 551-559.

     Keywords: perception, self-care

     A review of the research on perceptual functioning, body image dysfunction, and their relationship to performance in activities of daily living are presented and ideas for future studies are proposed.

304. Trombly, C. (Ed.) (1995). *Occupational therapy for physical dysfunction* (4th ed.). Baltimore: Williams & Wilkins.

     Keywords: cognition, motor, perception

     This classic textbook offers a number of chapters with varying degrees of discussion about the relationship between neuro-cognitive performance components and occupation. This book focuses on evaluation and remediation, as well as specific diagnoses resulting in cognitive and neurological problems.

305. Case-Smith, J., Allen, A. S., & Pratt, P. N. (Eds.) (1996). *Occupational therapy for children* (3rd ed.). St. Louis, MO: C. V. Mosby.

     Keywords: children, cognitive

Several chapters in this textbook provide information that contributes to our understanding of the relationship between neurological and cognitive performance components and occupation. Relevant to this theory area are chapters on development of hand skills, sensory integration, visual perception, feeding and oral skills, and prewriting and handwriting skills.

306. **Cornhill, H., & Case-Smith, J. (1996). Factors that relate to good and poor handwriting.** *Am J Occup Ther, 50(9), 732-739.*

Keywords: coordination, handwriting, perception

This study investigated the relationship between the performance components of eye-hand coordination, visuomotor integration, and in-hand manipulation and the occupation of handwriting. Test scores on the Motor Accuracy Test, Developmental Test of Visual-Motor Integration, Minnesota Handwriting Test, and two tests of in-hand manipulation were all significantly higher for the subjects with good handwriting than with poor handwriting.

307. **Pearson, S. (1996). An exploration of the effect of right homonymous hemianopia on engagement in occupation.** *Journal of Occupational Science, 3(1), 18-25.*

Keywords: activity, perception

A phenomenological approach was used to study the effect of right visual field loss on three people's engagement in occupation. A reduced level of activity satisfaction and decreased ability to engage in the occupations of driving, literacy, locating objects, and personal mobility were identified as relevant findings.

308. **Christiansen, C., & Baum, C. (Eds.) (1997).** *Occupational therapy: Enabling function and well-being* **(2nd ed.). Thorofare, NJ: SLACK Incorporated.**

Keywords: cognitive, motor, neuroscience

This comprehensive textbook offers three chapters relevant to this theory area: "Implementing Neuroscience Principles to Support Habilation and Recovery" by W. Dunn, "Movement Related Problems" by J.L. Poole, and "Meeting the Challenge of Cognitive Disabilities" by J.M. Duchek and B.C. Abreu.

309. **Ferguson, J. M., & Trombly, C. (1997). The effect of added-purpose and meaningful occupation on motor learning.** *Am J Occup Ther, 51, 508-513.*

Keywords: activity, motor

This experimental study showed that adults achieved increased motor learning in a situation where activities were perceived as purposeful and meaningful, compared to those engaged in a rote-learning task.

310. Katz, N., & Hartman-Maeir, A. (1997). Occupational performance and metacognition. *Canadian Journal of Occupational Therapy, 64*(2), 53-62.

Keywords: cognition, neuroscience

The concept of metacognition and its relationship to occupational performance, particularly in relation to clients with neurological dysfunctions, is explored. The authors stress the importance of integrating ideas about metacognition and occupational therapy theory.

311. Elm, D., Warren, S., & Madill, H. (1998). The effects of auditory stimuli on functional performance among cognitively impaired elderly. *Canadian Journal of Occupational Therapy, 65*(1), 30-36.

Keywords: sensory, motor

This study assessed functional performance skills of cognitively impaired elderly residents of a continuing care facility using the Assessment of Motor and Process Skills (AMPS). The residents were tested under three different auditory stimulus conditions: silence, conversation, and music. The results suggest that background music may have a negative effect on motor and process functional performance skills.

312. Gentile, A. M. (1998). Implicit and explicit processes during acquisition of functional skills. *Scandinavian Journal of Occupational Therapy, 5*(1), 7-16.

Keywords: learning, motor, rehabilitation

This article provides an explanation of implicit and explicit learning processes, and their application to the development of functional skills.

313. Parham, L. D. (1998). The relationship of sensory integrative development to achievement in elementary students: Four year longitudinal patterns. *Occupational Therapy Journal of Research, 18*(3), 105-127.

Keywords: learning, sensory integration

The longitudinal study described in this article investigated the relationship between perceptual abilities and achievement in math and reading in children 6 to 8 years old and again 4 years later. Participants included 32 children with learning disabilities and 35 children without. The results of the evaluation supported the study hypothesis that the relationship between sensory integrative factors and arithmetic skills was strong in the younger years but declined with age, whereas the opposite pattern was observed for reading skills.

314. Poole, J. L. (1998). Effect of apraxia on the ability to learn one-handed shoe tying. *Occupational Therapy Journal of Research,* 18(3), 99-104.

Keywords: apraxia, learning, perception

A study to examine the learning and retention ability of participants with left-hemisphere cardiovascular accident is described. Participants with apraxia were found to require significantly more trials to learn one-handed shoe tying and to retain the skill than the participants without apraxia.

315. Tse, D. W., & Spaulding, S. (1998). Review of motor control and motor learning: Implications for occupational therapy with individuals with Parkinson's disease. *Physical and Occupational Therapy in Geriatrics,* 15(3), 19-38.

Keywords: learning, motor

Principles of motor control and motor learning theories are reviewed and related to the occupational performance difficulties that people with Parkinson's disease experience. Implications for occupational therapy practice are discussed.

316. Cohen, H., & Reed, K. L. (1999). The historical development of neuroscience in physical rehabilitation. *Am J Occup Ther,* 50(7), 561-568.

Keywords: models, rehabilitation

The authors describe the parallel development of neuroscience research and neurorehabilitation theories relevant to occupational therapy, emphasizing common themes.

317. Dunbar, S. B. (1999). A child's occupational performance: Considerations of sensory processing and family context. *Am J Occup Ther,* 53(2), 231-235.

Keywords: cognition, perception, sensory

This article presents a discussion of the relationship between the effects of sensory processing dysfunction on cognition, sensory and motor development, and children's occupational performance in school and home environments.

318. Fleming, J., & Strong, J. (1999). A longitudinal study of self-awareness: Functional deficits underestimated by persons with brain injury. *Occupational Therapy Journal of Research,* 19(1), 3-17.

Keywords: cognition, self

A longitudinal study of 55 adults with traumatic brain injury investigated the areas of function for which they lacked self-awareness of their level of competency. The results indicated that self-awareness was most impaired for activities with a large cognitive and socio-emotional component and least impaired for basic activities of daily living, memory activities, and overt emotional responses.

---

319. Howell, D. (1999). Neuro-occupation: Linking sensory deprivation and self-care in the ICU patient. *Occupational Therapy in Health Care, 11*(4), 75-85.

Keywords: sensory, self-care

The emerging concept of neuro-occupation and its relationship to occupational performance is discussed in the context of self-care activities performed by patients in an intensive care setting. Implications for occupational therapy practice are identified.

---

320 Kramer, P., & Hinojosa, J. (Eds.) (1999). *Frames of reference for pediatric occupational therapists* (2nd ed.). Baltimore: Lippincott Williams & Wilkins.

Keywords: children, models

Pediatric occupational therapy theory and practice are structured around frames of reference with the focus on occupation. Section II includes chapters that explain the neurodevelopmental treatment, sensory integration, visual perception, and motor skill acquisition frames of reference.

---

321. Vakrat, R. Y., Katz, N., & Hoofien, D. (1999). Factors related to long-term performance in instrumental activities of daily living (IADL) of clients with brain damage: A retrospective follow-up study. *International Journal of Occupational Therapy, 8*(1), E3-E21.

Keywords: cognition, perception, self-care

A study to assess the relationship of objective and subjective variables to instrumental activity of daily living (IADL) performance of clients with brain damage is described. Results demonstrated that subjective variables of perception of cognitive deficits and acceptance of disability were stronger predictors of IADL performance than severity of brain damage. The authors propose that further theoretical conceptualizations and empirical studies are needed.

---

322. Way, M. (1999). Parasympathetic and sympathetic influences in neuro-occupation pertaining to play. *Occupational Therapy in Health Care, 12*(1), 71-86.

Keywords: neuroscience, perception, play

The author uses a neuro-occupation theoretical framework to explain the relationship between play and the autonomic nervous system.

323. Cooke, K. Z., Fisher, A. G., Mayberry, W., & Oakley, R. (2000). Differences in activities of daily living process skills of persons with and without Alzheimer's disease. *Occupational Therapy Journal of Research, 20*(2), 87-105.

Keywords: activity, cognition, self-care

The purpose of the study described in this article was to determine if persons with dementia of the Alzheimer type differed from nondisabled older persons in terms of the process skills that affect the performance of activities of daily living (ADL). The research concluded that the cognitive and physical impairments experienced by people with Alzheimer-type dementia negatively affect their ability to perform ADL.

324. Dunn, W. W. (2000). Habit: What's the brain got to do with it? *Occupational Therapy Journal of Research, 20*(Suppl), 6-20.

Keywords: cognition, habits, sensory

The author explores the concept of habits and presents a discussion of the neuroscience principles that explain their formation and maintenance.

325. Grieve, J. (2000). *Neuropsychology for occupational therapists* (2nd ed.). Oxford, England: Blackwell Science.

Keywords: activity, neuroscience

Although this book focuses primarily on basic neuroscience theory, the author discusses the effects of perceptual and cognitive impairment on occupational performance in Chapter 7, "Task Performance."

326. Katz, N., Hartman-Maeir, A., Ring, H., & Soroker, N. (2000). Relationships of cognitive performance and daily function of clients following right hemisphere stroke: Predictive and ecological validity of the LOTCA battery. *Occupational Therapy Journal of Research, 20*(1), 3-17.

Keywords: cognition, hemiplegia

The purpose of the study described in this article was to investigate the relationship between cognitive ability and task performance in people with right-hemisphere stroke. Results suggest that unilateral spatial neglect is the major predictor of functional outcomes. Cognitive skills were significantly related to activities of daily living task performance in subjects who did not experience neglect.

327. Schreiber, J., Sober, L., Banta, L., Glassbrenner, L., Haman, J., Mistry, N., et al. (2000). Application of motor learning principles with stroke survivors. *Occupational Therapy in Health Care, 13*(1), 23-44

Keywords: motor learning, stroke, environment

This study predicted that stroke survivors performing a purposeful task in a familiar environment would demonstrate greater retention and transfer of motor skills. The results were inconclusive.

328. Tseng, M. H., & Chow, S. M. (2000). Perceptual-motor function of school-age children with slow handwriting speed. *Am J Occup Ther, 54*(1), 83-88.

Keywords: handwriting, motor, sensory

This article describes a study of slow and normal speed handwriters ages 7 to 11 years. The objective was to enhance our understanding of the skills required for efficient handwriting. The authors concluded that upper-limb speed and dexterity skills are primary predictors of normal speed handwriters, whereas slow handwriters depend more on visual-sequential memory and visual-motor integration.

329. Weintrab, N., & Graham, S. (2000). The contribution of gender, orthographic, finger function, and visual-motor processes to the prediction of handwriting status. *Occupational Therapy Journal of Research, 20*(2), 121-140.

Keywords: coordination, handwriting, sensory

This study of fifth-grade students identified as good or poor handwriters concluded that visual-motor integration and finger functioning contributed significantly to the prediction of handwriting ability.

SOME IMPORTANT IDEAS ABOUT THE COGNITIVE-NEUROLOGICAL DETERMINANTS OF OCCUPATION:

- Occupational performance problems originating in the central nervous system (CNS) can be understood using theory from this area.
- This area of theory locates the source of occupational performance problems in the person.
- The cognitive-neurological determinants of occupation include cognitive functioning, motor control, sensation, and perception.
- It is important to distinguish between the mind and the central nervous system—both are responsible for thinking but use entirely different mechanisms.
- Occupational conceptual models help us to understand the cognitive or neurological requirements of occupation.
- There are a number of "named" theories in this theory area. A few examples include neurodevelopmental theory, cognitive disabilities, sensory integration, and proprioceptive neuromuscular facilitation.
- There are a number of authors whose names are typically associated with theories in this area, such as Allen, Ayres, Brunnstrom, Bobath, Carr and Shephard, and Rood.
- As our understanding of the brain and central nervous system has changed over time (since the mid-1960s), ideas about the cognitive neurological determinants of occupation have changed, and with them, ideas about how to treat cognitive and neurological deficits.
- Occupational therapists have contributed significantly to our understanding of the central nervous system, but only in recent years have they focused on the impact of CNS disorder for occupation.

HERE IS A PRACTICAL PROBLEM THAT MAY HELP TO RAISE SOME OF THE IMPORTANT IDEAS IN THE AREA OF COGNITIVE AND NEUROLOGICAL DETERMINANTS OF OCCUPATION:

Jane is an occupational therapist at a neurological hospital specializing in rehabilitation for people who have had strokes. Jane has 5 years' experience on a busy 18-bed stroke unit, with an average length of stay of 6 weeks. The rehabilitation team, of which Jane is a part, confers regularly. This team, composed of the OT, PT, nurses, neurologist, speech therapist, and social worker, provides integrated rehabilitation services. However, there is often considerable disagreement between providers as to the best approach to treatment. While the PT advocates Brunnstrom's stages of neurological recovery and proprioceptive neuromuscular facilitation, Jane herself prefers the neurodevelopmental approach. The other team members also have their own views about what works and what doesn't, and often raise ideas that don't fit with any of the approaches already mentioned. For example, the nurses often advocate stroking the hand to release spasticity, although there is some disagreement among them about whether to stroke the dorsum or the palm of the hand. In addition, Jane has been asked by a researcher to try some sensory integrative and cognitive rehabilitation techniques with several of her patients, as part of a study.

Recently, the discussions at team meetings have become the source of considerable tension and have threatened to hamper the functioning of the team. Jane examines occupational therapy's body of knowledge for principles and concepts that relate cognitive-neurological functioning to occupational performance.

12 THE SOCIO-CULTURAL DETERMINANTS OF OCCUPATION

Mary Ann McColl, PhD

Introduction

Some of the most basic and fundamental ideas in occupational therapy stem from this area of theory—that human beings reflect their social nature and their membership in a particular culture. Ideas that link occupation to values, beliefs, time, roles, habits, expectations, and norms are found classified under this heading. These are all socially mediated, socially constructed, or socially defined phenomena, and they all have considerable potential to affect occupation. Ideas about occupation that reflect how it is affected by relationships to primary (family) and secondary (friends, colleagues) groups in society would also be classified as socio-cultural determinants of occupation. So, too, would theory about how individuals internalize their culture, how beliefs and values affect occupation, and how rituals and customs shape occupation. Finally, the recent literature on spirituality and its effect on occupation is also considered under socio-cultural theory since religion, faith, and spiritual issues are all part of our internalized social and cultural ideology.

A Brief History of Socio-Cultural Theory

The field of occupational therapy began near the turn of the 20th century in response to a social movement called moral treatment. This movement had been afoot in the latter part of the previous century and was a reflection of the new humanism that characterized much of 20th century ideology. It emphasized the value and potential inherent in all human beings, even those with severe disabilities, such as mental illnesses. One corollary of the moral treatment approach was the idea that for individuals to function normally, the patterns of their life had to have some normality to them, including patterns of activity and rest. This idea is most memorably advanced for occupational therapists by the psychiatrist Adolf Meyer, who states:

> There are many rhythms which must be attuned to: the larger rhythms of night and day, of sleep and waking hours, of hunger and its gratification, and finally, the big four—

work and play and rest and sleep, which our organism must be able to balance even under difficulty. The only way to attain balance in all this is actual doing, actual practice, a program of wholesome living as the basis of wholesome feeling and thinking and fancy and interests.

Meyer, *Archives of Occupational Therapy*, 1922, 2

In this quote, Meyer introduces a number of the ideas that are prevalent in the early literature and that have come to form the foundation of modern occupational therapy:

- The idea of rhythms or patterns of activity (roles, habits)
- The idea that occupation is constituted of work (productivity), play (leisure), sleep, and rest (self-care)
- The notion of balance among productivity, leisure, and self-care
- The idea that occupational dysfunction can be remediated by occupation, or doing

Another of the founding members of the profession of occupational therapy, Eleanor Clarke-Slagle, developed these same ideas about the health-producing effect of activity taken in patterned and predictable ways. She became known for a therapeutic regimen called *habit-training*, whose primary objective was to provide meaningful occupation for hospital patients, thereby preventing them from spending their time in morbid and unhealthy ways (Slagle, 1924). These habits were constituted to simulate the cultural ideal of a productive lifestyle. The notion of normality and the pursuit of integration pervaded the literature of the period and extended through to 1950 (Nash, 1938; Pollack, 1938; Lockerbie, 1947).

The literature of the early 1940s is characterized by not only a recognition of the occupational nature of humans but also of their social nature. It was observed that social isolation and occupational dysfunction often went hand-in-hand, and one obvious way to counteract this was to pursue social therapeutic activity in groups. In this way, patients could not only learn from one another, but also benefit from the social contact of the group (Kindwall & McLean, 1941; Preston, 1942). In the 1960s, the idea of the therapeutic effects of the social environment was further developed. Using treatment approaches alternatively referred to as milieu therapy or the therapeutic community, therapists advanced the notion that occupational therapy goals could most effectively be achieved when the impact of the social environment was understood (Feuss, 1959; McNair, 1959; Bockoven, 1971; Opzoomer & McCordic, 1973).

The 1950s and 60s, however, also brought about a trend toward objectivity and empiricism that, while touted as the savior of the profession of occupational therapy, nearly led to the demise of some of our most fundamental ideas. The scientific revolution hit occupational therapy with all its reductionistic fervour, threatening the validity of many socio-cultural ideas like the use of time, the patterns of occupational activity, and the importance of values and beliefs. Despite a few excellent articles published in this period, the literature on socio-cultural theory is thin throughout the middle decades of the century (Dodson, 1959; Sanchez, 1964; Dyer, 1963).

In the early 1970s, the literature in occupational therapy began to recover some of the ideas that had been out of fashion in previous decades, with a particular emphasis on the relationship between work and leisure (Mielicke, 1967; Matsutsuyu, 1971; Maurer, 1971). Role theory, originating in psychology, became more prevalent in the occupational therapy literature, with particular references to Talcott-Parsons' notion of the *sick role* (Jones, 1974).

Geopolitical changes in the 1980s led to an increased awareness of culture in occupational therapy (Jamieson, 1985; Baptiste, 1988), including the range of values and behaviours of both therapist and client, which affect the performance of occupation. Also reflecting societal-level discussions of the role of religion in society and the relationship between faith and medicine, occupational therapists began to incorporate spirituality into their consciousness and their view of occupation (CAOT, 1981; Urbanowski & Vargo, 1994).

References

Baptiste, S. (1988). Chronic pain, activity and culture. *Canadian Journal of Occupational Therapy, 55,* 179-84

Bockoven, J. S. (1971). Legacy of moral treatment: 1890s to 1910. *Am J Occup Ther, 25,* 223-5.

Canadian Association of Occupational Therapists. (1981). *Guidelines for the client-centred practice of occupational therapy.* Ottawa, ON: Supply & Services Canada.

Dodson, D. W. (1959). Occupational therapy for what? A look at values. *Am J Occup Ther, 15,* 189.

Dyer, G. W. (1963). The fourth dimension of the patient's continuum. *Am J Occup Ther, 17,* 226-8.

Feuss, C. D. (1959). Occupational therapy in the therapeutic community. *Am J Occup Ther, 13,* 9-10.

Jamieson, M. (1985). The interaction of culture and learning: Implications for occupational therapy. *Canadian Journal of Occupational Therapy, 52,* 5-8

Jones, N. A. (1974). Occupational therapy and the aged. *Am J Occup Ther, 28,* 615-8.

Kindwall, J. A., & McLean, J. (1941). One hand for the ship. *Occupational Therapy and Rehabilitation, 20,* 223-9.

Lockerbie, L. (1947). Socialization through occupational therapy. *Occupational Therapy and Rehabilitation, 26,* 142-5.

Matsutsuyu, J. (1971). Occupational behaviour: A perspective on work and plany. *Am J Occup Ther, 25,* 291-3.

Maurer, P. (1971). Antecedents of work behaviour. *Am J Occup Ther, 25,* 295-7.

McNair, F. E. (1959). Milieu therapy. *Canadian Journal of Occupational Therapy, 26,* 93-98.

Mielicke, C. (1967). The meaning of work and use of leisure. *Canadian Journal of Occupational Therapy, 34,* 75-81.

Nash, J. B. (1938). The philosophy of busy-ness. *Occupational Therapy and Rehabilitation, 17,* 27-32

Opzoomer, A., & McCordic, L. (1973). Occupational therapy-a change of focus. *Canadian Journal of Occupational Therapy, 40,* 125-9.

Pollack, B. (1938). Aims and ideals of occupational therapy. *Occupational Therapy and Rehabilitation, 17,* 291-300.

Preston, G. H. (1942). Relating occupational therapy to reality. *Occupational Therapy and Rehabilitation, 21,* 17-24.

Sanchez, V. (1964). Relevance of cultural values for occupational therapy programs. *Am J Occup Ther, 18,* 1-5.

Slagle, E. C. (1924). A year's development of occupational therapy in New York state hospitals. *The Modern Hospital, 22,* 98-104.

Urbanowski, R. & Vargo, J. (1994). Spirituality, daily practice and the occupational performance model. *Canadian Journal of Occupational Therapy, 61,* 88-94.

KEYWORDS USED IN THIS CHAPTER			
Activity	Environment	Lifespan	Roles
Aging	Family	Meaning	Social
Balance	Groups	Models	Spirituality
Beliefs	Habit	Motivation	Time
Culture	Hierarchy	Philosophy	Values
Disability	History	Play	Work
Essence	Identity	Research	

Bibliographic Entries for Socio-Cultural Determinants of Occupation

330. Black, M. M. (1976). The occupational career. *Am J Occup Ther*, 30, 225-228.

Keyword: roles

The author suggests that occupational role is a determinant of health, reflecting an individual's adaptations to society. The concepts of role theory, occupational choice, and occupational career are discussed. Role acquisition throughout life is described as an occupational career.

331. Heard, C. (1977). Occupational role acquisition: A perspective on the chronically disabled. *Am J Occup Ther*, 31, 243-247.

Keywords: roles, social

Quality of life for people with chronic disabilities is conceptualized as being dependent upon the acquisition of new occupational roles. The article defines occupational role as consisting of daily activity, time use, contribution to society, and societal worth. This article presents the concept of role along with three critical points in the occupational role acquisition process.

332. Kielhofner, G. (1977). Temporal adaptation: A conceptual framework for occupational therapy. *Am J Occup Ther*, 31, 235-242.

Keyword: time

The concept of temporal adaptation is introduced as a useful concept from which human adaptation and dysfunction can be better understood. A temporal conceptual framework for occupational therapy evaluation and intervention is proposed, along with two case studies.

333. Meyer, A. (1977). The philosophy of occupational therapy. *Am J Occup Ther, 21*, 639-642.

Keywords: activity, balance, time

This is a commemorative reprint of the classic article that first appeared in 1922 in the *Archives of Occupational Therapy*. In it, Meyer laid out a template for the emerging profession of occupational therapy, including the ideas of a balance of work, rest and leisure, the inherent satisfaction of activity, and the use of time organized into healthy habits.

334. Versluys, H. (1980). The remediation of role disorders through focused group work. *Am J Occup Ther, 34*, 609-614.

Keywords: groups, roles

This article deals with two concepts in the socio-cultural area: roles and groups. Relevant concepts of role acquisition are reviewed, as well as the relationship between disability and its impact on personal role functions. Factors that contribute to the erosion of specific adult, occupational, family, and avocational roles are examined. Experiential groups are proposed as the method for addressing role acquisition.

335. Kielhofner, G., Barris, R., & Watts, J. H. (1982). Habits and habit dysfunction: A clinical perspective for psychosocial occupational therapy. *Occupational Therapy in Mental Health, 2*, 1-21.

Keywords: habits, hierarchy, models

The paper revives the concept of habits and interprets it within the context of the Model of Human Occupation. The authors explore principles of habit formation and conclude that habits integrate into higher-level systems while, at the same time, organize the lower-level systems. By meeting the demands of the environment and the volitional subsystem, habits (or patterned routines of behaviour) make adaptation possible.

336. Rogers, J. (1982). The spirit of independence: The evolution of a philosophy. *Am J Occup Ther, 36*, 709-715.

Keywords: philosophy, values

The concept of independence is central to occupational therapy. It is a defining feature of North American society, and its definition is heavily culturally mediated.

337. Vandenberg, B. (1982). Play in evolution, culture and individual adaptation: Implications for therapy. *Am J Occup Ther, 36*, 20-28.

Keywords: culture, play, environment

The author explores play and playfulness in a cultural context and derives a set of principles about the use of play in a therapeutic environment that are based on its social, cultural, and evolutionary significance.

338. Levine, R. (1984). The cultural aspects of home care delivery. *Am J Occup Ther, 38,* 734-738.

Keywords: culture, roles

This paper addresses the effects of values, goals, interest, roles, and habits as aspects of culture on occupational performance. It conceptualizes culture as a filter through which self-care, productivity, and leisure are viewed.

339. Jamieson, M. (1985). The interaction of culture and learning: Implications for occupational therapy. *Canadian Journal of Occupational Therapy, 52,* 5-8.

Keywords: culture, motivation

While acknowledging that culture affects many aspects of therapy, this article suggests that therapists have been less aware of the influence of culture on learning. Cultural variations in motivation style, cognitive style, human relational style, and social interaction are examined for their implications for occupational therapy service delivery.

340. Johnson, J. A. (1985). Wellness: Its myths, realities, and potential for occupational therapy. *Occupational Therapy in Health Care, 2,* 117-138.

Keywords: roles, values

The article advances the definition of wellness as a context for living, including the capacity for expressiveness, connectedness, recognition of values and roles, ability to care for oneself, and to master one's environment. Implications for occupational therapy include redefinition of both the client and the therapist role, as well as integration in the community.

341. Elliott, M. (1987). Occupational role performance and life satisfaction in elderly persons. *Occupational Therapy Journal of Research, 7,* 216-224.

Keywords: aging, roles, time

This study examined the relationship between life satisfaction and the number of meaningful roles performed in a sample of 112 community-dwelling elderly people. Based on the Model of Human Occupation, the study concludes that involvement in meaningful roles is essential to health and well-being.

342. Iannone, M. (1987). Cross-cultural investigation of occupational roles. *Occupational Therapy in Health Care, 4,* 93-101.

Keywords: culture, roles

This paper applies a cross-cultural perspective to occupational behaviour, with emphasis on the concept of occupational roles. Cultural implications for future theory development in occupational therapy are advanced.

---

343. Levine, R. E. (1987). Culture: A factor influencing the outcome of occupational therapy. *Occupational Therapy in Health Care, 4,* 3-16.

Keywords: culture, meaning

The author defines culture as a "blueprint for human behaviour, influencing individual thoughts and actions, and collectively influencing a particular society." Culture is examined as it affects the individual's perception of illness, therapy, and meaning in life.

---

344. Skawski, K. (1987). Ethnic/racial considerations in occupational therapy: A survey of the occupational therapy literature. *Occupational Therapy in Health Care, 4,* 37-48.

Keyword: culture

After examining the occupational therapy literature for cultural factors affecting occupational therapy, the author reports the results of a study of cultural sensitivity among occupational therapists and occupational therapy practice.

---

345. Baptiste, S. (1988). Chronic pain, activity and culture. *Canadian Journal of Occupational Therapy, 55,* 179-184.

Keywords: activity, culture, history

The author explores the connections between activity and its cultural interpretation and importance for individuals with chronic pain. The history of two central ideas is reviewed: culture and activity. Relationships between ethnic background, satisfaction with life roles, and activity levels are explored among people with chronic pain.

---

346. Krefting, L. H., & Krefting, D. V. (1991). Cultural influences on performance. In C. Christiansen & C. Baum (Eds.), *Occupational therapy: Overcoming human performance deficits* (pp. 100-122). Thorofare, NJ: SLACK Incorporated.

Keywords: culture, hierarchy

This article offers a definition of culture as concentric circles in which the individual participates, including family, peers, community, and nation. These spheres of culture each have an influence on the individual's occupational performance, and he or she, in turn, acts out culture through participation at each level.

347. Peloquin, S. (1991). Time as a commodity: Reflections and implications. *Am J Occup Ther, 45,* 147-154.

    Keywords: culture, time, values

    This article stems from the premise that occupation exists in time. It looks at images in the popular media as a way of understanding contemporary beliefs about time. It defines time as socially constructed and underlines the popular illusion that we control time. The author uses the example of a clock or watch as both a machine and a piece of jewelry to illustrate our views about time.

348. Rowles, G. (1991). Beyond performance: Being in place as a component of occupational therapy. *Am J Occup Ther, 45,* 265-271.

    Keywords: environment, habits, time

    Beyond knowing and doing, this article emphasizes being as an essential aspect of human occupational experience. The author advocates that greater attention is given to spatio-temporal patterns and rhythms in daily life.

349. Sparling, J. W. (1991). The cultural definition of the family. *Physical and Occupational Therapy in Pediatrics, 11,* 17-27.

    Keywords: culture, family, values

    The article begins with an exploration of demographic trends affecting the family. The author offers guidelines to help occupational and physical therapists to broaden their definition of family, and to assist in the identification of family priorities for intervention.

350. Branholm, I. (1992). Occupational role preferences and life satisfaction. *Occupational Therapy Journal of Research, 12,* 159-171.

    Keywords: lifespan, roles

    This is a report of a large empirical study of role performance in adults of varying ages. The study showed role preferences at different ages, ultimately describing a typical role career. Factor analysis identified meta-roles that were closely associated with satisfaction in different aspects of life.

351. Doble, S., & Magill-Evans, J. (1992). A model of social interaction to guide occupational therapy practice. *Canadian Journal of Occupational Therapy, 59,* 141-150.

    Keywords: models, social

    The article presents the Social Interaction Model as a framework for working with people with deficits in social interactions. The model conceptualizes social enactment skills as a function of sensory input, cognition, emotional state, volition, and interaction style.

352. Kielhofner, G. (1992). The group work model. In G. Kielhofner (Ed.), *Conceptual foundations of occupational therapy* (pp. 142-153). Philadelphia: F. A. Davis.

Keywords: groups, roles, values

This chapter discusses the group work model, originally proposed by Howe and Schwartzberg (1986). It describes the nature of therapeutic groups and the rationale for group work. It focuses on the manner and extent to which roles, values, habits, and meaning are determined in social groups.

353. Kinebanian, A., & Stomph, M. (1992). Cross-cultural occupational therapy: A critical reflection. *Am J Occup Ther, 46,* 752-757.

Keywords: activity, culture, values

This article offers the results of a survey of occupational therapists in the Netherlands on culturally mediated issues such as independence, purposeful activity, and roles. Further, it provides guidelines for occupational therapists for cross-cultural occupational therapy.

354. Van Deusen, J. (1993). Mary Reilly. In R. J. Miller & K. F. Walker (Eds.), *Perspectives on theory for the practice of occupational therapy* (pp. 155-178). Gaithersburg, MD: Aspen.

Keywords: models, roles, time

This chapter reviews the work of one of the most important contributors to theory in the socio-cultural area: Mary Reilly. The chapter discusses such ideas as temporal adaptation, occupational behaviour, occupational roles, and occupational dysfunction.

355. Wilcock, A. A. (1993). Biological and sociocultural aspects of occupation, health, and health promotion. *British Journal of Occupational Therapy, 56,* 200-203.

Keywords: essence, models

This article begins with the position that occupation is innate and essential to human life. Its purposes include survival, safety, health, and development. The author reviews seven approaches to promoting health through occupation, from the conventional medical approach to ecological approach.

356. Hallett, J., Zasler, N., Maurer, P., & Cash, S. (1994). Role change after traumatic brain injury in adults. *Am J Occup Ther, 48(3),* 241-246.

Keywords: brain damage, roles

The role checklist and semi-structured interviews were used to explore role change in 28 adults with brain injury living in the community. All reported role changes, with the majority identifying role losses. A discussion of the participants' perspectives and explanations for the changes contributes to occupational therapists' understanding of potential role change after traumatic brain injury.

---

357. Hutch, R. (1994). Family as vocation: An occupation on behalf of the generations. *Journal of Occupational Science (Australia), 1,* 11-20.

Keywords: family, work

Hutch compares and contrasts the popular philosophy of individualism with familism. He defines familism as a focus on children in terms of protecting, nurturing, and training. He suggests that familism is preferable to individualism both for the survival and the development of humans as individuals, and as societies and species.

---

358. Mirkopolous, C., & Evert, M. M. (1994). Cultural connections: A challenge unmet. *Canadian Journal of Occupational Therapy, 61,* 67-70.

Keywords: culture, values

The Canadian-American collaboration offers definitions for culture in the North American context. It includes concepts such as patterns of behaviour, shared history, ethnicity, and nationality. It suggests strategies for monitoring and overcoming incompatibility in cultural backgrounds between therapists and clients.

---

359. Urbanowski, R., & Vargo, J. (1994). Spirituality, daily practice, and the occupational performance model. *Canadian Journal of Occupational Therapy, 61,* 88-94.

Keywords: spirituality, meaning

This article defines spirituality as the experience of meaning in everyday life. It contrasts the idea of meaning in life with the somewhat grander notion of the meaning of life, and also with religiosity, meaning association with formal religion. The article also makes distinctions between spirituality and holism, ethics, and volition.

---

360. Paul, S. (1995). Culture and its influence on occupational therapy evaluation. *Canadian Journal of Occupational Therapy, 62,* 154-161.

Keyword: culture

This paper advances the ideas of culture-fair and culture-specific evaluation, and explores the potential for bias and misinterpretation that exists in a number of occupational therapy evaluations.

361. Christiansen, C. (1996). Three perspectives on balance in occupation. In R. Zemke & F. Clark (Eds.), *Occupational science: The evolving discipline* (pp. 441-451). Philadelphia: F. A. Davis.

Keywords: activity, balance, time

This chapter explores the idea of balance in occupation. Christiansen looks at time use and activity patterns as: perceived versus actual time use, chronobiological balance, and relationships among life tasks.

362. Gutman, S. A., & Napier-Klemic, J. (1996). The experience of head injury on the impairment of gender identity and role. *Am J Occup Ther, 50*(7), 533-544.

Keyword: role

This qualitative study explores the changes in perceived masculinity or femininity, intimate relationships, and gender roles of two men and two women at least 1 year post-injury. The men expressed more intense feelings of gender inadequacy than the women did, and the women reported resuming more pre-injury activities than the men did.

363. Yerxa, E. (1996). The social and psychological experience of having a disability: Implications for occupational therapists. In L. W. Pedretti (Ed.), *Occupational therapy: Practice skills for physical dysfunction* (pp. 253-274). St. Louis, MO: C. V. Mosby.

Keywords: disability, social

In this chapter, Yerxa reviews the values and beliefs of occupational therapists related to disability—holism, agency, and autonomy. She contrasts the outsider's view of disability with that of the insider, based on a number of autobiographical accounts. In addition to recommendations for society in general, she makes five recommendations for occupational therapists: doing away with the mind-body dichotomy, using occupation as therapy, changing values about mourning disability, focusing on the therapeutic relationship, and considering alternative models of practice.

364. Zemke, R., & Clark, F. (1996). *Occupational science: The evolving discipline*. Philadelphia: F. A. Davis.

Keywords: time, roles, values

This primer on occupational science offers a number of chapters on socio-cultural determinants of occupation, such as time, roles, meaning, and balance.

365. Clark, F. (1997). Reflections on the human as an occupational being: Biological need, tempo and temporality. *Journal of Occupational Science (Australia), 4*, 86-92.

Keywords: history, time

Clark looks to prehistoric occupations for a blueprint of the essence of occupation and the elements of occupation that are most compatible with health. She begins by defining humans as essentially occupational beings. She advances the notions of tempo (the pace of occupation) and temporality (the relationship of occupation to past, present, and future), and explores the intersection between these two concepts.

366. Engquist, D., Shortt-deGraff, M., Gliner, J., & Oltjenbruns, K. (1997). Occupational therapists' beliefs and practices with regard to spirituality and therapy. *Am J Occup Ther, 51*, 173-180.

Keywords: spirituality, values

This article presents a survey of 270 American occupational therapists about the concept of spirituality and its place in their practice. While 89% said they believed it belonged in occupational therapy's scope of practice, 67% said they only dealt with it if the client brought it up. A number of reasons for this are presented, including reimbursement issues, professional issues, and personal issues.

367. Fitzgerald, M., Mullavey-O'Byrne, C., & Clemson, L. (1997). Cultural issues from practice. *Australian Occupational Therapy Journal, 44*, 1-21.

Keywords: culture, roles

This paper incorporates the findings of two other surveys of occupational therapy students and practitioners with a review of the literature. It identifies seven issues for greater attention in the area of culture: professional values, family roles, communication patterns, social behaviors, gender roles, the sick role, and explanatory models.

368. Hasselkus, B. (1997). Meaning and occupation. In C. Christiansen & C. Baum (Eds.), *Occupational therapy: Enabling function and well-being* (2nd ed., pp. 362-377). Thorofare, NJ: SLACK Incorporated.

Keywords: culture, meaning, spirituality

In this chapter, Hasselkus talks about the visible and invisible aspects of occupation, or the performance and meaning components of occupation. She emphasizes the need to distinguish between the performance of occupation and the totality of the experience of occupation, which includes meaning. Meaning is related to culture and may involve aspects of ritual and spirituality.

369. Howard, B. S., & Howard, J. R. (1997). Occupation as spiritual activity. *Am J Occup Ther, 51*, 181-185.

Keywords: meaning, spirituality, time, work

In this article, the authors begin with the premise that disability interferes with the individual's search for meaning in life. They differentiate between spirituality and religion, as well as between the substantive and functional definitions of religion. They emphasize the importance of work and the use of time as two occupational therapy concepts that contribute to meaning in life.

---

370. **Kielhofner, G. (1997). The model of human occupation. In G. Kielhofner (Ed.), *Conceptual foundations of occupational therapy* (2nd ed.). Philadelphia: F. A. Davis.**

Keywords: habits, time, values

This chapter offers definitions and conceptual foundations for many of the ideas in the socio-cultural area, such as habits, values, and temporal adaptation. Although not all aspects of the Model of Human Occupation fit best in this theory area (e.g., environment, personal causation), much of the substance of this theory deals with determinants of occupation that are socially defined and mediated.

---

371. **Kroeker, P. T. (1997). Spirituality and occupational therapy in a secular culture. *Canadian Journal of Occupational Therapy, 64,* 122-126.**

Keyword: spirituality

Kroeker defines the context from contemporary occupational therapy as secular pluralism. The author maintains that the loss of shared spirituality is the price North American society has paid for scientific, material, and technical progress. It outlines skills required for spirituality in practice: patience, tolerance, sensitivity, awareness, and maturity.

---

372. **Ludwig, F. M. (1997). How routines facilitate well-being in older women. *Occupational Therapy International, 4,* 213-228.**

Keywords: habits, identity

This article posits a relationship between routines and a number of important health outcomes, such as activity level, balance, life satisfaction, and continuity. Based on the results of a small study of older women, it advances a model of the mechanism through which routines affect well-being, involving both the sense of self and relationships with others.

---

373. **McColl, M. A. (1997). Social support and occupation. In C. Christiansen & C. Baum (Eds.), *Occupational therapy: Enabling function and well-being.* (2nd ed., pp. 410-425). Thorofare, NJ: SLACK Incorporated.**

Keyword: social

This chapter offers an overview of the literature on social support, disability, and occupation, as well as recommendations for assessment and intervention. The chapter focuses on perceived support as an intrinsic factor affecting occupation.

---

374. Townsend, E. (1997). Inclusiveness: A community dimension of spirituality. *Canadian Journal of Occupational Therapy, 64,* 146-155.

Keywords: disability, spirituality

This article focuses on spiritual bonds that transcend the self and connect individuals with their communities. It maintains that an understanding of individual spirituality is inadequate to understand the full concept and that inclusiveness is an essential dimension of spirituality.

---

375. Collins, M. (1998). Occupational therapy and spirituality: Reflecting on quality of experience in therapeutic interventions. *British Journal of Occupational Therapy, 61,* 280-284.

Keywords: meaning, spirituality

Collins outlines five facets of experience: being, meaning, intention, expression, and spirituality. Quality of experience represents the interaction of the optimal levels of these five dimensions. The author encourages therapists to participate as co-creators of meaning in experience with clients.

---

376. Jones, D., Blair, S. E., Hartery, T., & Jones, R. K. (Eds.). (1998). *Sociology and occupational therapy: An integrated approach.* Edinburgh, Scotland: Churchill Livingstone.

Keyword: social

This book explores the theoretical basis of occupational therapy theory that comes from sociology. In particular, it focuses on concepts, such as role, gender, culture, family, and social interaction. It offers both depth and breadth of coverage of sociocultural concepts, and applies them directly to assessment and intervention in occupational therapy.

---

377. McGruder, J. (1998). Culture and other forms of human diversity on occupational therapy. In M. Neistadt, & E. B. Crepeau (Eds.), *Willard & Spackman's Occupational therapy* (9th ed., pp. 54-66). Philadelphia: Lippincott Raven.

Keyword: culture

This chapter defines culture using the metaphor of a lens through which individuals view the world and enact occupation. Culture is defined as shared, learned, durable, changeable, and invisible. It is not inherited, racial, ethnic, or language-specific. McGruder advocates for multicultural competence among occupational therapists.

378. Ribeiro, K., & Allens, J. (1998). Voluntarism as occupation. *Canadian Journal of Occupational Therapy, 65,* 279-285.

Keywords: identity, productivity

This article presents the results of a single case study exploring voluntary activity as an occupation. It highlights voluntary activity as a source of productivity and as a vehicle for the establishment of identity in an individual with mental illness.

379. Yerxa, E. (1998). Health and the human spirit of occupation. *Am J Occup Ther, 52,* 412-418.

Keywords: activity, balance

Yerxa contends that the human spirit for activity is actualized through occupation. She draws heavily on the work of Adolph Meyer and emphasizes the relationship between occupation and health. She explores a number of definitions of health in relationship to occupation.

380. Christiansen, C. (1999). Defining lives: Occupation as identity. An essay on competence, coherence and the creation of meaning. *Am J Occup Ther, 53,* 547-558.

Keywords: identity, meaning

This article asserts the idea that occupation is key to creating identity in humans. It is based on four propositions: that identity shapes relationships, that identity is tied to action and interpretation, that identity characterizes the central character in the self-narrative, and that identity is essential to well-being. Three aspects of identity are considered: the reflexive, interpersonal, and social aspects.

381. Clark, F. (2000). The concepts of habit and routine: A preliminary theoretical synthesis. *Occupational Therapy Journal of Research, 20,* 123-137.

Keywords: disability, habits

This article attempts to synthesize the literature to date on habits and routine with respect to three topics: definition, relationship to quality of life, and benefits to people with disabilities. Habits are believed to increase skill, decrease fatigue, and free attention. The author proposed five hypotheses about habits for future research.

382. Dunn, W. W. (2000). Habit. What's the brain got to do with it. *Occupational Therapy Journal of Research, 20,* 6-20.

Keywords: habits, motivation

This article advances the idea of a habit continuum, from habit impoverishment to habit domination. At the balance point is habit utility. Dunn reviews neuroscience principles underlying the existence of habits, such as attention thresholds, modulation, motivation, and sensation seeking and avoiding.

383. McColl, M. A. (2000). Spirit, occupation and disability. *Canadian Journal of Occupational Therapy, 67,* 217-228.

Keywords: *disability, spirituality*

This article looks at definitions associated with spirituality and how they have been understood in occupational therapy literature. It also addresses the potential importance of spirituality in the lives of people with disabilities and explores some of the reasons for this. Finally, the article synthesizes occupational therapy approaches for intervention in the area of spirituality.

384. Rogers, J. C. (2000). Habits: Do we practice what we preach? *Occupational Therapy Journal of Research, 20,* 119-122.

Keyword: *habit*

This article elaborates the ideas generated at a conference on habits: the nature of habits, relationship between skill training and habit training, the context of habits, dysfunction in habits, and the potential for boredom as a result of an excess of habit.

385. Tickle-Degnen, L., & Trombly, C. (2000). The concept of habit: A research synthesis. *Occupational Therapy Journal of Research, 20,* 138-143.

Keywords: *habits, research*

This article summarizes a research agenda for the study of habits. Research questions fall into three general categories: specification and definition, descriptive and relational questions, and intervention approaches.

386. Whiteford, G., & Wilcock, A. A. (2000). Cultural relativism: Occupation and independence reconsidered. *Canadian Journal of Occupational Therapy, 67,* 324-336.

Keywords: *culture, meaning*

This is a study of occupational therapy students used to highlight the importance of culture for understanding socially constructed concepts, such as occupation and independence. These two ideas are central to occupational therapy and, yet, have been shown in this study to be culturally sensitive.

SOME IMPORTANT IDEAS ABOUT THE SOCIO-CULTURAL DETERMINANTS OF OCCUPATION:

- ✖ This area of theory locates the source of occupational performance problems in the person.
- ✖ In particular, this area of theory focuses on internalized socially constructed phenomena and their effects on occupation.
- ✖ The socio-cultural determinants of occupation include concepts like values, roles, habits, use of time, beliefs, and social support.
- ✖ These concepts are usually acquired by individuals through the process of socialization and social adaptation.
- ✖ It is important to distinguish between:

  (a)internalized aspects of society and culture, versus

  (b) the impact of the external realities of society and culture, specifically the social and cultural environments.
- ✖ Occupational conceptual models help us to understand how the messages we have internalized from our families; communities; and social, cultural, and ethnic groups affect what we do.
- ✖ Many parts of the Model of Human Occupation may be classified in this theory area, such as ideas about values, interests, roles, and habits. There are other aspects of the model that make more sense in other theory areas.
- ✖ Group therapy simulates the impact of groups in our socialization and social adaptation; therefore, it is important to understand how groups function and how individuals function within groups.
- ✖ Socially constructed phenomena have no external reality, only internalized and shared definitions. For example, we have internalized ideas about time: when we should get up in the morning and go to bed at night, how much time it is appropriate to spend on the telephone, how many minutes late it is tolerable to be for an appointment, etc.
- ✖ Socially constructed phenomena, such as time, differ from person to person and certainly from culture to culture. In order to effectively apply the socio-cultural model of practice, it is essential to have an understanding of the internalized message by which an individual is governed.
- ✖ Although anthropologists, sociologists, and social psychologists have added much to our understanding of social and cultural aspects of people and occupations, much of this theory area arises directly out of the work of the founders of occupational therapy, such as Meyer and Slagle.
- ✖ More recent contributions come from Reilly, Kielhofner, and their associates.

HERE IS A PRACTICAL PROBLEM THAT MAY HELP TO RAISE SOME OF THE
IMPORTANT IDEAS IN THE AREA OF SOCIO-CULTURAL DETERMINANTS OF
OCCUPATION:

Theresa is an occupational therapist who works in an exclusive private mental health facility in Long Beach, CA. About a year ago, unbeknownst to the press, a well-known media personality was admitted to this facility in a state of acute withdrawal and agitation. From the day of her admission, Theresa began to work with this patient and determined that the source of her problem was the lack of structure or meaning in her daily activities and routines. The two worked intensively together over a 6-week period to:

✖ unravel her roles

✖ determine the privileges and constraints of those roles

✖ understand what she found meaning in

✖ uncover her underlying value system and its origins in her family and culture

✖ restructure her use of time to add meaning and purpose to her life

Despite the secrecy around this admission, upon discharge, this famous personality was quite open with the press about her "breakdown" and effusive in her praise of the care she had received at the clinic. As a result, Theresa and the other three members of the team were asked to appear with her on a television talk show to discuss the nature of their treatment and the factors that had contributed to its success.

In preparation for her appearance, Theresa traced the development of socio-cultural theory from the late 19th century to present times and the expression of these ideas in occupational therapy.

13 | THE ENVIRONMENTAL DETERMINANTS OF OCCUPATION

Mary Law, PhD

Introduction

The environmental area of occupational therapy theory focuses on factors within the physical, social, cultural, and institutional environments that affect occupation. As stated earlier in the book, using environmental theory leads to a structural analysis of occupational issues. Change in occupation is facilitated through change or accommodation of the environment, rather than the person. Basic theories that contribute to our understanding in this area come from many disciplines, including anthropology, ecology, geography, sociology, political science, and economics. For the purposes of this book, environment is those contexts and situations that occur outside the individual and elicit responses in them. Different environments include cultural, physical, economic, institutional, and social environments. Environments can facilitate or limit participation in everyday occupations. The transactional relationship between persons, the occupations they choose to do, and in the environments in which they live, work, and play ultimately determines the person's occupational performance (Law et al., 1996).

A Brief History of the Environmental Determinants of Occupation

In the early decades of the occupational therapy profession from 1910 until 1930, there was very little written specifically about the environment or environmental determinants of occupation. The only references to environment within the occupational therapy literature at this time discussed the need for healthy hospital environments. During the 1930s, although there were no specific writings about environmental theory, the literature discussed how a patient relates to the environment and how occupational therapy could provide environments that were conducive to recovery and the promotion of skill development. It was also during this decade that occupational therapists began outpatient clinics as a means to assist patients in their readjustment to the community environment.

The decade of the 1940s focused primarily on the rehabilitation of soldiers. In the literature of the era, the mental aspects of rehabilitation and the importance of looking at the whole person within the physical and social environment were stressed. Discussion focused on how occupational therapists could modify the environment to influence a person's behaviour. The increased emphasis on the environment continued through the 1950s, but with the influence of the medical model, references to the environment always separated it into the physical and social dimensions. An exception to this influence was an article by O'Reilly (1954) in which she discussed person-environment interaction and the need to fit the patient into the environment so that their community life could be resumed with minimal stress. Other authors continued to talk about the effects of the environment on human behaviour, particularly the effects of colour, and the effects of the physical environment on older adults.

From 1960 until 1975, the literature on the specific application of environmental theory to different areas of occupational therapy practice increased substantially. There was a growth in the use of assistance devices and other environmental adaptations to promote independence for persons with disabilities. Occupational therapists were part of the creation of *prosthetic environments* in the institutions for older adults as a means of minimizing the disabling factors that cause stress. The role of the environments in influencing behaviour in the area of mental health and the development of a community-oriented conceptual approach to treatment in this area was emphasized. As well, enrichment of the environment was seen as a way to modify behaviour in pediatrics. Occupational therapists also began to view the environment as having many interactive variables affecting clients, and the need for persons to alter or improve the environment was discussed in order to maximize independence. In the early 1970s, occupational therapists had an increased interest in the occupational therapist's role of relating to minimizing architectural barriers. The importance of the environment in the development of play and other skills in children was articulated. A seminal article by Dunning (1972) discussed environmental occupational therapy, in which the person is viewed within his or her total environmental context.

References

Dunning, G. (1972). Environmental occupational therapy. *Am J Occup Ther, 26*, 292-8.

Law, M., Cooper, B., Strong, S., Stewart, D., Rigby, P., & Letts, L. (1996). The Person-Environment-Occupation Model: A transactive approach to occupational performance. *Canadian Journal of Occupational Therapy, 63*, 9-23.

O'Reilly, J. A. (1954). Occupational therapy in the management of traumatic disabilities. *Canadian Journal of Occupational Therapy, 21*, 75-80.

KEYWORDS USED IN THIS CHAPTER			
Activity	Culture	Personal causation	Support
Adolescent	Disability	Philosophy	Systems
Aging	Ecological	Physical	Technology
Assistive devices	Independent living	Psychological	Time
Beliefs	Institutional	Rehabilitation	Work
Children	Meaning	Sensory	
Community	Models	Social	

Bibliographic Entries for Environmental Determinants of Occupation

387. Laurence, M. K., & Banks, S. I. (1978). Milieu therapy and the elderly: A role for the occupational therapist consultant. *Canadian Journal of Occupational Therapy, 45*, 171-173.

Keywords: aging, institutional, support

This article presents the conceptual framework of milieu therapy as a treatment tool for institutionalized elderly persons. The underlying principles of a therapeutic community are first outlined. The role of the occupational therapist as a consultant is described in terms of "treating" the staff and organization within the nursing home milieu. The occupational therapist works with ward staff to help them understand and assimilate the occupational therapy objective of restoring the residents to an optimum level of physical, mental, social, and vocational independence. The concept of the occupational therapist as a "change agent" in establishing a milieu therapy program in a nursing home is considered to be important in redefining his or her role and facilitating the staff's growth in a supportive environment.

388. Parent, L. (1978). Effects of a low-stimulus environment on behavior. *Am J Occup Ther, 32*, 19-25.

Keywords: institutional, meaning, sensory

Psychological studies related to sensory and perceptual deprivations, immobilization, and isolation provide a body of literature that describes behavioural deficits occurring in experimental low-stimulus and meaningless environments. Specific hospital environments analogous to those used in the sensory deprivation experiments can also be used to identify patients who may be at high risk for maladaptive behavioural change. The studies offer extensive experimental evidence to support the occupational therapy theory that a variety of meaningful tasks and stimuli are necessary to support the hospitalized person's adaptive behaviour.

389. Kannegieter, R. (1980). Environmental interactions in psychiatric OT—Some inferences. *Am J Occup Ther, 34*, 715-720.

Keywords: institutional, psychological

Five inferences drawn from research studies in the social sciences on the assessment of psychiatric ward atmospheres are presented as a frame of reference for psychiatric occupational therapists. The studies, based on a model stating that behaviour results from the interaction of person and environment, suggest procedures for increasing successful treatment outcomes in OT. Such procedures include matching patients and staff to behavioural settings according to individual response traits and the development of programs emphasizing such variables as spontaneity, autonomy, and involvement.

390. **Keilhofner, G. (1981). An ethnographic study of deinstitutionalized adults: The community setting and daily occupations.** *Occupational Therapy Journal of Research, 1, 125-142.*

Keywords: community, institutional

The article presents the results of a 3-year ethnographic study of 69 deinstitutionalized developmentally handicapped adults. The results are analyzed according to two environments in which these individuals functioned: the residential facility and other community environments. The study presents many original quotes to illustrate the fact that deinstitutionalized individuals cannot be considered fully integrated in their communities but rather participating in a less formal institution.

391. **Barris, R. (1982). Environmental interactions: An extension of the model of occupation.** *Canadian Journal of Occupational Therapy, 36, 637-644.*

Keywords: personal causation, roles

The author explores the idea of incorporating environmental themes into the model of occupation, which broadens the concept of occupational performance. An individual's relationship to the environment is discussed in three areas: (1) properties of the environment that influence personal causation and the development of interests and values; (2) the demands of the environment for performance and their influence on the development of roles, habits, and skills; and (3) factors affecting a person's participation in an expanding range of settings.

392. **Howe, M. C., & Briggs, A. K. (1982). Ecological systems model for occupational therapy.** *Am J Occup Ther, 36, 322-327.*

Keyword: systems

The authors propose that the ecological systems model can conceptualize the theoretical and practice goals of occupational therapy. Ecology is the study of the relationship between organisms and their environment. States of health and illness are viewed as reflections of ecological adaptation. A human being is viewed as an open system participating as part of the ecosystem. Humans and the environment are interconnected and shape each other. Function and dysfunction are defined in terms of the clients' effectiveness in achieving their goals for quality of life in their interactions with the ecosystem. The implications for practice are discussed.

393. **Kiernat, J. (1982). Environment: The hidden modality.** *Physical and Occupational Therapy in Geriatrics, 2, 3-12.*

Keywords: aging, rehabilitation

This article focuses on the idea that special attention should be paid to environmental considerations when trying to change the behaviour of an older client. The article discusses the use of environment as a treatment modality. It is concluded that the environment must be viewed as an integral part of any rehabilitation program and that therapists must assess the client's psychosocial and physical environment and use this information as another modality in order to facilitate independence.

394. Kirchman, M. M., Reichenback, V., & Giambalvo, B. (1982). Preventive activities and services for the well elderly. *Am J Occup Ther, 36,* 236-242.

Keywords: aging, community, support

This article describes a joint service and research project established for a healthy elderly population in the United States. It demonstrates the value of providing a support system through intervention which helps the elderly remain in the community and improves life satisfaction. Interviews were conducted before and after an occupational therapy program, and the results showed significant improvement in four important areas: economic resources, social resources, life satisfaction, and general affect.

395. Reed, K. L. (1984). Generic models. In K. L. Reed (Ed.), *Models of practice in occupational therapy.* **(pp. 97-154). Baltimore: Williams & Wilkins.**

Keyword: models

The environment is considered in varying degrees in each of five models, selected by the author because each explains the values and beliefs of occupational therapy. In the occupational behaviour model, the environment is seen as something to be mastered, altered, and improved. The integrated theory of occupational therapy considers the external, socio-cultural environment as an influence on pre- and postnatal development, and as a factor that can feed or hinder development. The environment, including physical space and culture, interacts with human processes in an increasingly complex manner through a person's lifespan in the human development through occupation model. In the model of human occupation, the environment, which includes the physical, social, and cultural settings, interacts with an open human system, resulting in occupation. Environmental needs or demands serve as the inputs in the adaptive response model systems approach. The author describes each of these models in terms of their frames of reference, assumptions, and major concepts, and provides an analysis and critique of each model.

396. Frieden, L., & Cole, J. A. (1985). Independence: The ultimate goal of rehabilitation for spinal cord-injured persons. *Am J Occup Ther, 39,* 734-739.

Keywords: community, independent living

The role of independent living programs in overcoming the barriers that prohibit quality of life for disabled persons are described. Ideas are given on how occupational therapists can operationalize the concepts of the independent living movement to help disabled people live independently. Using a broad theoretical framework of occupation allows therapists to consider independence as a process that emphasizes self-direction and choices. The role of the occupational therapist, thus, expands beyond focusing on physical skills, thereby helping clients learn to overcome barriers and develop workable solutions to problems within a community context.

---

397. Bachelder, J. (1985). Independent living programs: Bridges from hospital to community. *Occupational Therapy in Health Care, 2,* 99-107.

Keywords: community, independent living

A brief history of the independent living movement is first presented in this article, followed by a discussion of the three models of independent living and the services they provide. Because occupational therapy has always advocated the independence of the client, the issues of independent living and the transition from hospitalization to independence are seen as important issues that need to be addressed. The three common independent living programs discussed are independent living centres, transitional living programs, and residential independent living programs.

---

398. Cooper, B. (1985). A model for implementing colour contrast in the environment of the elderly. *Am J Occup Ther, 39,* 253-258.

Keywords: aging, sensory

Much has been written on the use of colour as a functional facilitator in the environment of the elderly, but little information is available on how to implement it. This paper restates the main age-acquired visual defects, critically examines the literature on the use of environmental colour, and proposes a model that incorporates the factors that enhance visual clarity and contrast. Implicit in the application of colour to enhance vision is a clear understanding of structure-function relationship in the environment.

---

399. Barris, R. (1986). Activity: The interface between person and environment. *Physical and Occupational Therapy in Geriatrics, 5,* 39-45.

Keywords: activity, aging

This paper combines two bodies of literature, aging and the environment and aging and activity, to explore the relationship of the older person to his or her environment through activity. Barris describes factors in the environment such as culture, resources, and number of people, which can significantly influence a person's activity. It concludes with recommendations for enhancing control, variety, and interest.

400. Mosey, A. C. (1986). Environment. In A. C. Mosey (Ed.), *Psychosocial components of occupational therapy* (pp. 171-189). New York: Raven Press.

Keywords: culture, physical, social

   In this chapter, the author discusses the importance of considering a person's past, present, and future environments in evaluation and intervention in psychosocial occupational therapy. Examples of how occupational therapists can utilize the environment in practice are given, and the cultural, social, and physical environments are described in detail. Culture is defined and described, and the factors that lead to various cultural differences are explored. The relationships between the issues of health and illness and the cultural environment are also explored. The author explores four cross-cultural social factors that affect the social environment. Finally, seven physical environmental factors that have immediate impact on the individual's psychosocial capacity are highlighted.

401. Mosey, A. C. (1986). The nonhuman environment. In A. C. Mosey (Ed.), *Psychosocial components of occupational therapy* (pp. 193-198). New York: Raven Press.

Keyword: physical

   Two aspects of the nonhuman environment, which includes the physical environment, are described in this chapter: the nature of the nonhuman environment, and its use as a tool in occupational therapy. The capacity of the nonhuman environment to facilitate development and act as a source of anxiety and tension are described. The nonhuman environment can also be used as a tool. In this capacity, it can pose a challenge for mastery, facilitate occupational performance, and assist in the development of performance components. Examples of the use of the nonhuman environment as a tool in occupational therapy are given.

402. Washburn, M. G. (1986). Designing environments for the elderly. *Occupational Therapy in Health Care, 2, 17-25.*

Keywords: aging, institutional

   This article discusses planning living environments for the elderly and the unique role that occupational therapy can play. The author suggests that there is a definite role for occupational therapy in the designing of retirement centres because of the profession's philosophy of maximizing health through active living and the occupational therapist's knowledge and understanding of the aging process. It is concluded that because designing living environments for the elderly requires consideration of all aspects of residents' characteristics and functional abilities, it is important for occupational therapy to be involved in the architectural design as well as planning of programs for the environments of the elderly.

---

403. Rader, E. G. (1987). Ergonomics, occupational therapy and computers. *Occupational Therapy in Health Care, 3,* 43-53.

Keywords: ergonomics, work

This article discusses the basic ergonomic design principles for computer workstations. The arrangement of the work stations is discussed in relation to the physical and psychological adaptations that must be made in an automated work environment. The author suggests that the occupational therapist, who has knowledge of ergonomics as well as training in job analysis, work simplification methods, biomechanics, psychological and behavioural adaptation patterns, and sensory feedback mechanisms, will be better prepared to help the user-patient to adjust to his or her work station and achieve greater productivity.

---

404. Robinson L. (1987). Patient compliance in occupational therapy home health programs: Sociocultural considerations. *Occupational Therapy in Health Care, 4(1),* 127-37.

Keyword: community

In this article, the author stresses the importance of awareness and understanding the many factors that affect a person's participation in the treatment process in home care settings. Four main factors related to compliance to occupational therapy treatment plans by individuals are discussed, including poor comprehension, social and environmental influences, characteristics of the regimen, and relationship between patient and health care provider. A three-step compliance model in occupational therapy home care programs is then outlined.

---

405. Llorens, L. A. (1989). Health care system models and occupational therapy. *Occupational Therapy in Health Care, 5,* 25-37.

Keywords: models, systems

Five prevailing theoretical models of occupational therapy practice are discussed in this article, as are four future scenarios in health care system models. The models of occupational therapy that are presented include the occupational behaviour model, the human occupation model, the occupational performance model, the developmental model, and the adaptive response model. The author discusses the importance of the interaction between the five models and four systems. It is concluded that occupational therapy should function as an open system that is flexible and able to maintain itself in a changing environment.

---

406. Christenson, M. A. (1990). Adaptations of the physical environment to compensate for sensory changes. *Physical and Occupational Therapy in Geriatrics, 8,* 3-30.

Keywords: adaptation, aging, sensory

This article deals with age-related changes in vision, hearing, taste, smell, touch, and kinaesthetic systems that occur in older adults. Recommendations are provided for environmental adaptation and modifications that may compensate for the changes in each of these systems. It is suggested that any physical setting can be designed and modified to allow individuals to operate at their maximum potential. Therapists are encouraged to strive for and plan environments that stimulate and respond to the sensory needs of the older person.

---

407. Christiansen, M. A. (1990) Designing for the older person by addressing environmental attributes. *Physical and Occupational Therapy in Geriatrics, 3,* 31-48.

Keywords: aging, competence, sensory

This paper discusses the importance of designing living environments for older adults that promote optimal adaptation levels, which are balances between the person's competence and environmental demand. The author encourages the occupational therapist to use the environment in her or his overall treatment plan. The environment is conceived as encompassing both physical and social components. The 12 key attributes of the living environment of older adults are described in terms of their effects on the occupants' well-being and occupational performance: comfort, legibility, privacy, accessibility, adaptability, meaning, control, density, security, dignity, aesthetics, and sensory stimulation. Suggestions for optimal designs are made.

---

408. Jongbloed, L., & Crichton, A. (1990). A new definition of disability: Implications for rehabilitation practice and social policy. *Canadian Journal of Occupational Therapy, 57,* 32-37.

Keywords: disability, rehabilitation

The authors describe a shift toward a socio-political definition of disability from an individualistic one and outline the implications of this shift for rehabilitation services in Canada. Because the socio-political definition of disability stresses the importance of environmental barriers in determining disability outcomes, rehabilitation professionals need to pay greater heed to environmental contexts and view clients as consumers of a service. While some progress has been made in terms of shelter and transportation policies since 1981, little headway has been made in employment and income maintenance policies. Barriers affecting socio-political policy and rehabilitation service development are discussed. The authors make several recommendations for working under the new framework.

---

409. Law, M. (1991). The environment: A focus for occupational therapy. *Canadian Journal of Occupational Therapy, 58,* 171-179.

Keywords: disability, physical

The author explores how several factors, including the physical environment, production of space, classification of individuals based on norms, labeling disability as deviance, power imbalances between health care professionals and clients, and increased bureaucracy in institutions, have led to disabling environments that limit occupation for persons with disabilities. Ideas about occupation are explored, and an approach to occupational therapy intervention to change disabling environments, with the active participation of people with disabilities, is proposed.

410. Boschen, K., & Krane, N. (1992). A history of the independent living movement in Canada. *Canadian Journal of Rehabilitation, 6,* 79-88.

Keywords: independent living, rehabilitation

The authors provide a brief historical account of the major events and factors leading to the formation of the independent living (IL) movement in North America. They suggest that social forces, such as politics, economics, and medical advances, have influenced the establishment of the IL movement. An evolution of the rehabilitation paradigm based on the medical model is given. Five main factors leading to the IL movement are described, including rejection of the medical model, deinstitutionalization, normalization, civil rights, and consumerism, and sports. The authors also describe American and Canadian legislation that supports IL and provide definitions of IL and IL centres. The history and development of the two main Canadian organizations involved in IL are also discussed.

411. Cooper, B., & Hasselkus, B. (1992). Independent living and the physical environment: Aspects that matter to residents. *Canadian Journal of Occupational Therapy, 59,* 6-15.

Keywords: independent living

In this paper, qualitative data from seven clients with disabilities, interviewed to gain their perspective on the issues involved in independent community living, is presented. The six most consistently identified themes are presented and discussed as parts of a working model of environmental control (MEC). Control, found to be the central construct of the MEC, and other control factors are discussed. Eight case studies that support the idea that personal control is central to independent living are briefly described. The authors suggest further testing and refinement of the model before its use in guiding clinical interventions.

412. Crist, P. A. H., & Stoffel, V. C. (1992). The Americans with Disabilities Act of 1990 and employees with mental impairments: Personal efficacy and the environment. *Am J Occup Ther, 46,* 434-443.

Keywords: psychological, work

In order to describe the implementation of the Americans with Disabilities Act (ADA) in occupational therapy and its effect on people with mental health problems in the work place, aspects of the ADA and its implications for people with mental health impairments are discussed in this article. The authors describe Bandura's theory of self-efficacy and strategies to facilitate increased self-efficacy of workers. In addition, four environmental aspects related to the employment of people with mental health impairments and the implications for occupational therapy are discussed. Examples of the effects on occupational therapy as a result of the implementation of the ADA are also discussed.

413. Hagedorn, R. (1992). Occupational therapy models. In R. Hagedorn (Ed.), *Occupational therapy: Foundations for practice—Models, frames of reference and core skills* (pp. 57-69). Edinburgh, Scotland: Churchill Livingstone.

Keyword: models

Three models (the model of human occupation, the adaptation through occupations model, and the adaptive skills model) are described in terms of their primary assumptions, patient-therapist relationships, applications, and techniques. In the model of human occupation, the environment is described in terms of the influence of press on occupational behaviour. In the adaptation through occupations model, the influence of the environmental context and content on occupational performance is described. The environment, in the adaptive skills model, consists of cultural, social, and physical aspects that provide the context of occupational performance.

414. Kalscheur, J. A. (1992). Benefits of the Americans with Disabilities Act of 1990 for children and adolescents with disabilities. *Am J Occup Ther, 46,* 419-426.

Keywords: children, disability

This article discusses the philosophical framework of occupational therapy, stating that functional independence requires an interactive relationship between the person and the environment. The relationship of the ADA to pediatric occupational therapy practice is discussed. An environment-centred model of practice, compatible with the philosophies of the Americans with Disabilities Act, is proposed, and three case examples of its application in the social, physical, and temporal environments are presented.

415. Reed, K. L., & Sanderson, S. N. (1992). Models of occupational therapy being explored and discarded. In K. L. Reed & S. N. Sanderson (Eds.), *Concepts of occupational therapy* (3rd ed., pp. 53-71). Baltimore: Williams & Wilkins.

Keyword: models

In this chapter, two occupational therapy models that include the environment are compared with others that do not. The first is the model of human occupation, which suggests that occupation be studied as an open system interacting with the environment. In this model, the person is changed by, and can change, the environment. The second model discussed is part of a health service continuum model. Accommodation programs that deal with environmentally related problems encompass this model.

416. Reed, K. L., & Sanderson, S. N. (1992). Toward a theoretical model of occupational therapy. In K. L. Reed & S. N. Sanderson (Eds.), *Concepts of occupational therapy* (3rd ed., pp. 87-93). Baltimore: Williams & Wilkins.

Keywords: adaptation, models

The authors present 11 key assumptions and their underlying concepts in the form of a proposed conceptual model of occupational therapy. This model includes the concepts of adaptation and the environment, while the organization of occupations is stressed. The environment is conceptualized as three separate, overlapping aspects, which include the physical, psychobiological, and sociocultural environments. Occupational therapy can either enable the individual to adapt to the environment or allow the environment to adapt to an individual through the use of occupations. Principles of practice based on the proposed model are presented.

417. Law, M., & Dunn, W. (1993). Perspectives on understanding and changing the environments of children with disabilities. *Physical and Occupational Therapy in Pediatrics, 13*, 1-16.

Keywords: children, disability

Compared to children without disabilities, restrictive physical environments, normative classification, and the power of the health disciplines have led to environmental constraints restricting the participation by children with disabilities in communities. The authors discuss the efficacy of historical solutions, including the biomedical model, to these disabling environments and conclude that they have had little effect on improving the conditions for children with disabilities. A shift toward the emerging socio-political model of disability is proposed, which not only considers disability as a problem in the interaction between the environment and the person but also stresses the use of social policies to change the environment. The principles and implications for practice of a socio-political planning model are presented.

418. Dunn, W., Brown, C., & McGuigan, A. (1994). The ecology of human performance: A framework for considering the effect of context. *Am J Occup Ther, 48*, 595-607.

Keywords: ecological, model

The ecology of human performance (EHP) is proposed as a model for elucidating the relationships between persons and their contexts, and the effects of this relationship on human behaviour and occupational performance. The contexts include the temporal, physical, social, and cultural domains. Use of the EHP for occupational therapy intervention is outlined by means of case examples, and directions for future work are proposed.

419. Griswold, L. A. S. (1994). Ethnographic analysis: A study of classroom environments. *Am J Occup Ther, 48, 397-402.*

Keywords: children, institutional

This article presents the results of ethnographic analytical observations in eight elementary school classrooms from two school districts in New Hampshire. The purpose of this ethnographic study was to analyse the structural environments and cultures of classrooms in order to help occupational therapists determine their roles, and appropriate interventions for, particular classroom environments. The author distinguished three categories, each with several subcategories that are organized into a classroom observation guide, which can be used to guide assessments of specific classrooms. An analysis of two different classrooms using this guide is outlined, and implications for occupational therapy practice are highlighted.

420. Polatajko, H. J. (1994). Dreams, dilemmas, and decisions for occupational therapy practice in a new millennium: A Canadian perspective. *Am J Occup Ther, 48, 590-594.*

Keyword: disability

The author presents her vision of a world: (1.) That is free of handicap, not just by rehabilitation, but by the creation of supportive environments to enable people to live with dignity; (2.) where occupational therapy will begin to fully realize and utilize the full potential of occupation; and (3.) where occupational therapy will become a profession focused on enabling occupation through purposeful activity to prevent handicap, rather than on focusing on reducing impairment alone. Occupational performance is presented as the result of an ideal fit between the person, environment, and occupation.

421. Dow, P. W., & Rees, N. P. (1995). High-technology adaptations to overcome disability. In C. A. Trombly (Ed.), *Occupational therapy for physical dysfunction* (4th ed., pp. 611-643). Baltimore: Williams & Wilkins.

Keywords: assistive devices, technology

Descriptions of several low- and high-technology devices to enable independence in occupational performance are described in this paper. These include computers, augmentative and alternative communication devices, and environmental control units. The ways assistive technology enhances occupational performance are discussed, and an assessment process for assistive technology is presented. A case study applying the assistive technology process is offered.

422. Grady, A. P. (1995). Building inclusive community: A challenge for occupational therapy. 1994 Eleanor Clarke Slagle Lecture. *Am J Occup Ther, 49, 300-310.*

Keywords: community, disability

In this talk, ideas about inclusion, community, relationships between the environment and community, transactions between the person and environment, and the interactions between a person's past and present experiences and future hopes are presented. Current ideas about disability and influences on participation are also discussed. A challenge to occupational therapists to develop more interactive models of practice is presented. The author also presents an expanded view of the environment category in the spatiotemporal adaptation theory, previously developed in conjunction with Gilfoyle and Moore. A model for environment-person relationships is shown as a spiralling continuum. The paper highlights outstanding challenges for profession, and concludes with strategies for occupational therapy to promote collaborative models of consumer-driven, community-based practice based on an interactive communication model.

---

423. **Hagedorn, R. (1995). Environment. In R. Hagedorn (Ed.),** *Occupational therapy: Perspectives and processes* **(pp. 93-101). Edinburgh, Scotland: Churchill Livingstone.**

Keyword: ecological

The author highlights the growing recognition in occupational therapy of the physical, social, and cultural environments and their influences on the individual. In particular, it is noted that the socio-ecological-developmental view of persons is gaining currency in the occupational therapy literature. Definitions of the environment in general, and the cultural, social, and physical environments in particular, are given. The ability of the environment to enhance or impede occupational performance is discussed, and the importance and methods of environmental analysis highlighted. The author also discusses two types of environmental adaptation aimed at improving performance as part of occupational therapy.

---

424. **Trombly, C. A. (1995). Theoretical foundations for practice. In C. A. Trombly (Ed.),** *Occupational therapy for physical dysfunction* **(4th ed., pp. 15-27). Baltimore: Williams & Wilkins.**

Keyword: physical

The hierarchical model and five major conceptual models of practice that guide occupational therapy for physical dysfunction are described. Contributions of the physical and social environments to the person's occupation, and therapeutic interventions that include environmental modifications are highlighted.

---

425. **Brayman, S. J. (1996). Managing the occupational environment of managed care.** *Am J Occup Ther, 50,* **442-446.**

Keywords: adaptation, institutional

The health care revolution in the United States has resulted in managed care environments and lead to the reorganization of hospitals and other health care institutes. The author discusses the observations arising from focus group discussions at a university teaching hospital that were designed to understand the effects of these changes on the occupational performance on the hospital's workers. The occupational adaptation model, which describes the interaction between the person and the environment, is used to explain the effects of the physical, social, and cultural components of the occupational environment on the practitioner attempting to adjust to the changing health care system.

---

426. Craddock, J. (1996). Responses of the occupational therapy profession to the perspective of the disability movement. Part 2. *British Journal of Occupational Therapy, 59(2), 73-78.*

Keywords: disability, philosophy

In this second of a two-part literature review, the author describes the responses of the occupational therapy profession in North America and the United Kingdom to the changing perspective of the disability movement. A social model of disability defines disability as a problem resulting from the interaction of the environment and the person, as contrasted to the medical model, which locates the problem of disability within the person. The importance of disabling environmental factors is highlighted in the social model, and the implications for occupational therapy philosophy and practice resulting from its adoption are described. The author predicts a clarification of occupational therapy's conceptual base and changed professional role if the profession embraces the social model of disability. A possible three-step intervention approach is outlined, and research that addresses how the social and medical models may be used by occupational therapy to guide practice is described.

---

427. Fidler, G. S. (1996). Life-style performance: From profile to conceptual model. *Am J Occup Ther, 50, 139-147.*

Keywords: activity, models

The life-style performance model is presented by the author as a framework for understanding a person's activities within her or his environment and is conceptualized by the interpersonal, societal, cultural, physical, and temporal domains. This model stresses the role of the environment in its ability to maximize individual performance to the extent that it optimizes some or all of the different characteristics of the person and activity. Four domains of individual performance, including self-care and maintenance, intrinsic gratification, social contribution, and interpersonal relationships are addressed. A framework for applying the model in occupational therapy prevention or remediation is outlined.

---

428. Law, M., Cooper, B., Strong, S., Stewart, D., Rigby, P., & Letts, L. (1996). The person-environment-occupation model: A transactive approach to occupational performance. *Canadian Journal of Occupational Therapy, 63, 9-23.*

Keyword: models

The authors propose a transactive person-environment-occupation model of occupational performance derived from, and influenced by, environment-behaviour theories and the Canadian guidelines for occupational therapy practice. The model evolved in response to changing views of the relationship between persons and their environments, including the recognition that occupational performance may be described as the result of dynamic relationships between persons, their environments, and their occupations and roles. Major assumptions of the model, the person-environment-occupation fit, and implications for practice are discussed. The model is illustrated with a case example.

---

429. Orr, C., & Schkade, J. (1996). The impact of the classroom environment on defining function in school-based practice. *Am J Occup Ther, 51, 64-69.*

Keywords: children, institutional, roles

Although school environment has been shown to influence function among children in schools, decisions are still based on deficits in component skills. In order to study the extent that occupational therapists consider context in their interventions, a study was carried out to determine the extent to which occupational therapists in one school district addressed student role demands in their interventions. Using the model of student role adaptation, 22 special education teachers identified the demands of children 3 to 6 years of age. The results show that the five occupational therapists that participated in this study addressed the classroom environmental demands identified by the special education teachers when designing their interventions.

---

430. Christiansen, C., & Baum, C. M. (1997). Person-environment occupational performance: A conceptual model for practice. In C. Christiansen, & C. Baum (Eds.), *Occupational therapy: Enabling function and well-being* (2nd ed., pp. 46-70). Thorofare, NJ: SLACK Incorporated.

Keywords: models, systems

The authors present the person-environment occupational performance model based on systems theory in which the person, as an open system, is depicted in interaction with the environment. In this model, occupational choice and performance are influenced by intrinsic and extrinsic factors. Extrinsic factors are described as the cultural and physical environment, social support, and societal factors. An application of the model in occupational therapy assessment and intervention is described, and illustrated with a case comparison.

---

431. Corcoran, M., & Gitlin, L. (1997). The role of the physical environment in occupational performance. In C. Christiansen & C. Baum (Eds.), *Occupational therapy: Enabling function and well-being* (2nd ed., pp. 336-360). Thorofare, NJ: SLACK Incorporated.

Keywords: models, physical

The key aspects of the physical environment as they relate to and affect occupational performance are described. The interactions between human capabilities and the physical environment, as well as between physical and sociocultural factors, are portrayed as complex transactions that influence occupational performance. Concluding this chapter are discussions on assessments of the physical environment and enhancement of occupational performance within six therapeutic frameworks.

---

432. Finlayson, M., & Edwards, J. (1997). **Evolving health environments and occupational therapy: Definitions, descriptions and opportunities.** *British Journal of Occupational Therapy, 60,* 456-460.

Keyword: institutional

The authors document a shift in thinking about illness and wellness toward primary health care, which includes a greater focus on health promotion. Definitions and descriptions of several important, overlapping concepts guiding this reform are given. Examples are given to examine the links between occupational therapy and the new health environments as defined by these concepts, as well as how occupational therapists are working in these environments.

---

433. Kielhofner, G. (1997). **The model of human occupation.** In G. Kielhofner (Ed.), *Conceptual foundations of occupational therapy* (2nd ed., pp. 187-217). Philadelphia: F. A. Davis.

Keywords: models, systems

In this chapter, the author describes the model of human occupation as one that explains occupational behaviour and discusses the subsystems and factors that influence it. The environment is described as comprising physical and social elements that provide affordance or press in both function and dysfunction. Seven general therapeutic principles are presented, in which the environment is seen as the only tool occupational therapists have to change in order to support or encourage change in the human system. Applications of the model by assessments, data interpretation, intervention methods, and program development are presented. The types of research focused on the MOHO are briefly described, and a suggestion for future research is made.

---

434. Kielhofner, G. (1997). **The spatiotemporal adaptation model.** In G. Kielhofner (Ed.), *Conceptual foundations of occupational therapy* (2nd ed., pp. 271-287). Philadelphia: F. A. Davis.

Keywords: models, time

The author provides a brief description of the revised version of the spatiotemporal adaptation model, originally proposed by Gilfoyle, Grady, and Moore (1981). The interdisciplinary base is described, and the influence of occupational therapy literature on childhood play on the newest version of the model is highlighted. The environment is one of four key variables described in the model's theoretical arguments. Therapeutic intervention approaches are described, and the environment is seen as an element that may require structuring to promote adaptation in the child. Assessment techniques and treatment using a *spiral process* are briefly described.

---

435. **Law, M., Cooper, B. A., Strong, S., Stewart, D., Rigby, D., & Letts, L. (1997). Theoretical contexts for the practice of occupational therapy. In C. Christiansen & C. Baum (Eds.), *Occupational therapy: Enabling function and well-being* (2nd ed., pp. 72-102). Thorofare, NJ: SLACK Incorporated.**

Keyword: models

The key theoretical concepts underlying occupational therapy practice and its views of the person, environment, and occupation are described. The authors outline 10 models from the environment-behaviour studies literature and their potential use in occupational therapy. The key concepts and theoretical bases for six occupational therapy models of practice that emphasize the person-environment-occupation relationship are then described, and the implications for practice are highlighted.

---

436. **Law, M., Polatajko, H., Baptiste, S., & Townsend, E. (1997). Core concepts of occupational therapy. In E. Townsend (Ed.), *Enabling occupation: An occupational therapy perspective*. Ottawa, ON: CAOT ACE.**

Keywords: beliefs, models

The authors present the occupational therapy values and beliefs that guide occupational therapy practice in enabling occupation. A new model to guide OT practice, the Canadian model of occupational performance (CMOP), is presented. This model represents the dynamic relationship between persons, the environment, and occupation. Definitions of these three elements are given, and the environment includes cultural, institutional, physical, and social aspects. Occupational performance is described as the interaction of the person, environment, and occupation. This chapter concludes with a discussion of client-centred practice with individuals, groups, organizations, and others.

---

437. **Bain, B. K. (1998). Assistive technology in occupational therapy. In M. E. Neistadt, & E. B. Crepeau (Eds.), *Willard & Spackman's occupational therapy* (9th ed., pp. 498-517). Philadelphia: Lippincott Raven.**

Keywords: assistive devices, technology

The author first highlights and describes the occupational frames of reference that guide assistive technology rehabilitation. A consumer-task-environment-device model is then proposed to frame evaluation of consumers for assistive technology devices. A description of currently available assistive technology, including the categories of switches, control interfaces and input devices, augmentative and alternative communication, and powered mobility and environmental controls is presented.

---

438. Baum, C., & Law, M. (1998). Community health: A responsibility, an opportunity, and a fit for occupational therapy. *Am J Occup Ther, 52,* 7-10.

Keyword: community

In response to society's changing definition of health, the authors encourage the profession to shift its thinking from a biomedical to a sociomedical context, and to take an active role in building healthy communities. In this new context, occupational therapists can help change the environment and social policy rather than the person. Several ways in which occupational therapists can meet these challenges are discussed, along with new competencies that the authors feel are essential to practice in a rapidly evolving health system. In response to this change, occupational therapists are encouraged to remain client-centred in a multidisciplinary community approach that enhances clients' function in restorative, as well as preventive, health maintenance programs.

---

439. Dunn, W., McClain, L. H., Brown, C., & Youngstrom, M. J. (1998). The ecology of human performance. In M. E. Neistadt & E. B. Crepeau (Eds.), *Willard & Spackman's occupational therapy* (9th ed., pp. 531-534). Philadelphia: Lippincott Raven.

Keyword: ecological

The authors highlight the role of ecology, or the interaction between persons and their contexts in influencing behaviour and task performance. The underlying assumptions and definitions of the components of the ecology of human performance (EHP) is presented in this paper, and the environment is comprised of physical, social, and cultural aspects. Five intervention strategies within the EHP, which focus either on the person's abilities, tasks, or environment and their applications for practice are presented.

---

440. Holm, M. B., Rogers, J. C., & Stone, R. G. (1998). Person-task-environment interventions: A decision-making guide. In M. E. Neistadt & E. B. Crepeau (Eds.), *Willard & Spackman's occupational therapy* (9th ed., pp. 471-498). Philadelphia: Lippincott Raven.

Keywords: activity, ecological

The authors begin with a review of ecological models that emphasize the person-task-environment (PTE) transactions and describe the components of these transactions. The utility of PTE transactions is discussed in the context of function and dysfunction in occupational therapy. Two major evaluation and intervention approaches, the top-down and bottom-up, are then discussed in terms of their advantages and disadvantages. A guide for systematic clinical decision-making is presented, followed by a discussion on formulating target outcomes and intervention.

---

441. Kellegrew, D. H. (1998). Creating opportunities for occupation: An intervention to promote the self-care independence of young children with special needs. *Am J Occup Ther, 52*(6), 457-465.

Keywords: children, disability, independence

A study exploring the relationship between opportunities for occupation and the skill performance of three children ages 28 to 32 months with special needs is described. The results indicate that there was a relationship between the structure of the environment and the ability, and eventual independence, of self-care in two of the children. Further research to investigate the association between environmental opportunities and occupation for children with disabilities is proposed.

---

442. Kielhofner, G., & Barrett, L. (1998). The model of human occupation. In M. E. Neistadt & E. B. Crepeau (Eds.), *Willard & Spackman's occupational therapy* (9th ed., pp. 527-529). Philadelphia: Lippincott Raven.

Keywords: models, systems

The model of human occupation is presented as a framework for understanding a client and his or her strengths and challenges, and for selecting and implementing occupation therapy intervention. The author states that the MOHO utilizes a systems view for understanding the person as an occupational being within an environmental context which influences occupational behaviour. A description of the subsystems contributing to occupational behaviour, and the role of the physical and social environment in affording opportunity and press, is followed by suggestions on applying the model to practice.

---

443. McColl, M. A. (1998). What we need to know to practice occupational therapy in the community. *Am J Occup Ther, 52*, 11-18.

Keywords: community, models

This article examines the community as an environment for occupational therapy practice and considers three models for delivering service in a community context: client-centred, community-based rehabilitation, and independent living. Each has specific requirements in terms of theoretical support, and the relationship between theory and practice is explored.

---

444. Strong, S. (1998). Meaningful work in supportive environments: Experiences with the recovery process. *Am J Occup Ther, 52*, 31-38.

Keywords: psychological, work

The author uses a qualitative, ethnographic approach to identify the major themes underlying the meaning of work for 12 persons with persistent and considerable psychiatric disabilities who worked at an affirmative business in Hamilton, Ontario. The ability of work to facilitate change in a person's self-concept and self-efficacy was also explored. This change process is depicted as one involving the interaction of the person, work environment, and external environmental factors. Implications of the study for occupational therapy are presented.

445. Sussenberger, B. B. (1998). Socioeconomic factors and their influence on occupational performance. In M. E. Neistadt & E. B. Crepeau (Eds.), *Willard & Spackman's occupational therapy* (9th ed., pp. 67-79). Philadelphia: Lippincott Raven.

Keyword: social

Socio-economic factors are highlighted as the source of inequities in material resources and opportunities in society. The authors describe how these imbalances impact a person's occupational performance in the areas of education, work, leisure, and self-care. An examination of the U.S. health care system is presented in the context of the larger political economy. Impacts of economic environment on occupational therapy practice, and suggestions for client-centred practice in an increasingly challenging environment, are examined. The paper concludes with four vignettes showing the influence of socioeconomic factors on occupational performance.

446. Backhouse, M., & Rodger, S. (1999). The transition from school to employment for young people with acquired brain injury: Parent and student perceptions. *Australian Occupational Therapy Journal, 46*(3), 99-109.

Keywords: institutional, support, work

This study explores the perceptions of young people with brain injury and their parents toward the transition from school to employment. The findings indicated that most of the participants experienced lack of support from allied health and educational professionals in meeting obstacles related to school and work transitions.

447. Law, M., Haight, M., Milroy, B., Willms, D., Stewart, D., & Rosenbaum, P. (1999). Environmental factors affecting the occupations of children with physical disabilities. *Journal of Occupational Science, 6*, 102-110.

Keywords: children, disability

This paper presents the results of a qualitative study that examined the environmental factors limiting the participation of children with disabilities in daily occupations. Through focus groups and interviews, parents of 22 families that had a disabled child, between the ages of 3 and 12 years participated. The results identified attitudinal and institutional barriers as the most significant environmental factors limiting participation. Significant themes for changing disabling environments identified by the parents included the desire for: more control, increased use of inclusion to change attitudes, more flexible bureaucracies, and change in how society views normality.

---

448. **Strong, S., Rigby, P., Stewart, D., Law, M., Letts, L., & Cooper, B. (1999). Application of the person-environment-occupation model: A practical tool.** *Canadian Journal of Occupational Therapy, 66,* 122-133.

Keyword: models

Applications of the person-environment-occupation (PEO) model and its relationship to the Canadian model of occupational therapy are presented in this paper. Through three case examples, the authors illustrate how the PEO model may be used in planning, assessment, evaluation, and communication of occupational performance interventions.

---

449. **Hemmingsson, H., & Borell, L. (2000). Accommodation needs and student-environment fit in upper secondary schools for students with severe physical disabilities.** *Canadian Journal of Occupational Therapy, 67,* 162-172.

Keywords: adolescent, disability, institutional

The authors report the results of a study looking at the accommodation needs of 48 students with physical disabilities attending one of four specially adapted upper secondary schools in Sweden. A semi-structured school setting interview was used to assess the students' accommodation needs. Several areas for further accommodation were identified. The authors conclude with recommendations for improving the student-environment fit.

---

450. **Prellwitz, M., & Tamm, M. (2000). How children with restricted mobility perceive their school environment.** *Scandinavian Journal of Occupational Therapy, 7(4),* 165-173.

Keywords: children, disability, institutional

Findings based on the content analysis of qualitative interviews conducted with 10 students with restricted mobility suggest that physical and social environment issues contributed to their experience of disability. It is concluded that changes to these environments could increase the students' opportunities to participate in both teaching and social activities.

451. Tamm, M., & Skar, L. (2000). How I play: Roles and relations in the play situations of children with restricted mobility. *Scandinavian Journal of Occupational Therapy, 7*(4), 174-182.

Keywords: children, disability, play

The study described in this paper used a grounded theory approach to explore the play of children ages 6 to 12 years with restricted mobility. Discussion of the findings, which indicated that most of the children played alone or with an adult, was based on Mead's theory of identity development and Bronfenbrenner's theory of developmental ecology.

SOME IMPORTANT IDEAS ABOUT THE ENVIRONMENTAL DETERMINANTS OF OCCUPATION:

- This area of theory locates the source of occupational performance problems entirely outside of the person (i.e., in the environment).

- The environment consists of physical, social, cultural, institutional, political, and many other aspects.

- The environment may be considered as three concentric spheres, with the most proximal representing the immediate family and the most distal representing society as a whole.

- Occupational conceptual models help us to understand how the environment acts on individuals and their occupation.

- Occupational models of practice focus exclusively on change in the environment; therefore, therapeutic interventions must address the problem solely in the environment.

- Environmental models of practice do not seek to bring about any change in the person.

- Home assessments, ergonomics, and universal design are all aspects of the model of practice referring to the physical environment.

- Aids and adaptations that are proximal to the individual, and which alter function for him or her specifically, should be classified as one of the person models (physical, cognitive-neurological, psychological-emotional, or socio-cultural).

- Adaptations and modifications that are distal to the individual and that may benefit a number of people with similar problems should be classified under the environmental model of practice.

HERE IS A PRACTICAL PROBLEM THAT MAY HELP TO RAISE SOME OF THE
IMPORTANT IDEAS IN THE AREA OF ENVIRONMENTAL DETERMINANTS OF
OCCUPATION:

Trevor is an occupational therapist working on a vocational unit in a large rehabilitation hospital. People are usually referred to Trevor by their primary occupational therapist if there is a need for major vocational evaluation and readjustment following rehabilitation. Margot has been referred to Trevor to assess her ability to return to her previous employment as a bank teller. Margot was in a car accident several months ago, in which she sustained a mild brain injury and a moderate physical disability. She has worked for the bank for 17 years and would like to return as soon as she is able.

Working together with Margot, Trevor concluded that she would be unable to return to the job of a drive-through teller that she had held previously due to architectural barriers, the demands for speed and accuracy on the job, and the need for intense contact with the public. He contacted the bank's human resources department on Margot's behalf to inquire about what her options might be. The personnel officer at the bank, while helpful and cooperative, outlined only two options:

- ✖ To take disability benefits, which would represent a 23% loss of income

- ✖ To be trained for another less demanding position, which would represent a decrease in grade and salary

On the advice of counsel, Margot decided to pursue legal action, seeking retraining and reinstatement at her previous salary grade. In the course of this suit, Trevor was subpoenaed to provide testimony regarding the environmental conditions required for Margot to return to work. To clarify the situation in his own mind, Trevor set out to do a comprehensive evaluation of the environmental factors influencing Margot's return to work.

14 | THERAPEUTIC PROCESSES TO CHANGE OCCUPATION

Mary Ann McColl, PhD

To this point, we have talked about the first two basic principles of occupational therapy: that occupation is essential to human beings, and that occupation changes in response to internal and external demands. This chapter deals with the third principle of occupational therapy—occupational therapists can use occupation as a therapeutic medium to promote health and well-being. It shows how theory discussed so far helps occupational therapists know what to do.

As outlined in the first chapter, occupational therapists have three ways of using occupation therapeutically: remediation, compensation, and advocacy:

- ✖ *Remediation* means changing some aspect of the person, in order to fix a problem in occupational performance.

- ✖ *Compensation* means working around a problem, by using other components of the individual or the environment to improve occupation.

- ✖ *Advocacy* means acting on behalf of a client to pursue a change in the environment that will ultimately enhance occupation.

Remediation

As discussed in the first chapter, and as illustrated in Table 1-2, remediation is directed at person factors (i.e., the physical, psychological-emotional, cognitive-neurological, or socio-cultural aspects of the person). Furthermore, remediation tends to be associated with two types of change: development and adaptation.

- ✖ *Development*—remediation may be used to promote change that is intrinsically programmed, such as structuring the therapeutic medium or environment to offer the "just-right challenge" in the hope of stimulating the development of a new skill. In this case, the new skill that is sought is believed to be the next logical progression of a developmental process.

- ✖ *Adaptation*—remediation can also be used to promote adaptation by offering therapeutic activities that simulate an environmental challenge and promote exploratory behaviour and ultimately mastery. In this case, the interaction with the environment acts as a feedback loop that shapes purposeful responses into adaptive behaviour.

In both of these cases, remediation is used to bring about change in person factors:

* Changes in strength, range of motion, or endurance (physical determinants of occupation)

* Changes of thoughts or feelings (psychological-emotional determinants)

* Changes in cognitive or neurological processing (cognitive-neurological determinants)

* Changes in socially or culturally defined constructs like values, roles, or habits (socio-cultural)

Compensation

Compensation can be directed at both person factors and environment factors. In other words, when a therapist seeks to improve occupation by working around a problem, it may be necessary to recruit skills and resources from both the person and the environment in order to do so. Compensation typically occurs when a therapist judges that it is more efficient or more appropriate to work around a problem than to tackle it head on and try to "fix" it. Some people would say that compensation should only be considered when remediation has been attempted and failed, while others say that compensation should be considered from the outset.

Those in the former group would assert that a therapist's job is to make every effort to bring the person to his or her optimal functional level in all areas of human performance: physical, psychological-emotional, cognitive-neurological, and socio-cultural. They would contend that the first principle of therapy is to restore function to the person. Those in the latter group would say that every therapeutic strategy has to be evaluated on its merits for a particular person in a particular context. If in some cases it proves more effective to compensate than to remediate, then time and effort that could be spent on something more meaningful to the individual should not be wasted on remediation. The following example illustrates this idea:

> Joe has quadriplegia. At 19, he was hurt in a sports accident, and now, after surgery and recovery, he has been transferred to rehabilitation to begin preparing for life in the community. One of the main things on Joe's mind is how he will support himself, since his former job as an audio/electronics technician does not seem practical to him given his impaired hand function. He has always loved electronics, particularly audio equipment, and wishes to remain involved.

For the therapist committed to remediation before compensation, therapy would consist of exercises and activities aimed at restoring Joe's hand function to its highest level. Splints and adaptive devices might be used, with the objective of increasing dexterity and fine-motor performance to allow Joe to return to his vocation. Compensation would only be considered after an appropriate amount of time and effort had been devoted to remediation and it was determined that success was not achievable. Both Joe and his therapist realized that further efforts at remediation would produce diminishing returns, and the likelihood was small of achieving enough hand function to return to a career in electronics.

For the therapist who favoured compensation as a therapeutic approach, the emphasis would not be on restoring Joe's hand function, but rather on finding ways of working around the impaired hand function to allow him to have a productive occupation in the field of electronics. They might begin with an inventory of other skills and resources that Joe has at his disposal. What skills, equipment, approaches, or assistance could be marshaled to make Joe's productive goal possible? How could Joe approach the issue of having a job in the electronics field, other than the most obvious approach of doing the same thing he had done before? Needless to say, compensation can involve a great deal of creativity and resourcefulness, and it requires a mindset that does not dismiss options too readily or block suggestions before they are fully explored.

Neither of these two approaches is right all the time. Judgment is required to correctly ascertain how to balance these two therapeutic approaches: when to push for more functional restoration, when to pursue other options, or when to look outside the person for the solutions to his or her problems. This judgment accounts for a therapist's knowledge of both the personal and environmental determinants of occupation (in other words, the theory discussed in the previous chapters).

Advocacy

When the origin of a problem is clearly located outside the individual, then the way to change that problem is to accommodate for it (see Chapter 8). The therapeutic strategy associated with problems located outside the individual is advocacy. Advocacy is an approach to therapy wherein the therapist takes the part of his or her client and seeks change in the environment to benefit the client. Advocacy can have one client as its focus, or a group of clients who share the same problem. In all cases, the problem is an aspect of the environment that either directly impedes occupation or that fails to adequately support occupation. Successful advocacy depends on a thorough understanding of how the environment affects occupation (i.e., it depends on the theory discussed in the last chapter).

> When Joe was ready to move from the rehabilitation centre into the community, there were no apartments available for rent that would meet his needs. He required an apartment that was fully wheelchair accessible and within the limited budget afforded by his insurance settlement. Furthermore, Joe required transportation in the community that was wheelchair accessible and flexible enough to accommodate his work and social schedules.

From the perspective of compensation, Joe and his therapist would have to problem-solve methods of adapting an apartment to meet Joe's needs and, where possible, altering Joe's methods for doing things to suit the limitations of the apartment he could afford. Similarly, on the transportation issue, the compensatory approach would seek to make changes in Joe's existing transportation arrangements to accommodate his needs. The emphasis in both cases would be focused on Joe himself and his personal needs and resources.

From the advocacy perspective, Joe's issues would be seen in the larger socio-political context of people living in the community with a disability, and solutions would be sought that addressed these issues on a system-wide basis rather than on an individual basis. In other words, housing issues would be addressed in the context of the availability of accessible housing for all people with disabilities in a particular community, as well as for Joe as an individual. Similarly, transportation issues would be addressed in terms of making the public

Table 14-1	Therapeutic Processes to Change Occupation		
	REMEDIATION	**COMPENSATION**	**ADVOCACY**
Physical Determinants of Occupation	✖ Exercise ✖ Adapted activity ✖ Splinting	✖ Work simplification ✖ Energy conservation ✖ Assistive devices	✖ Physical accessibility
Psychological-Emotional	✖ Skills training ✖ Coping strategies ✖ Stress management	✖ Task adaptation	✖ Public education ✖ Community inclusion
Cognitive-Neurological	✖ Cognitive rehab ✖ Sensory integrative therapy	✖ Compensary techniques for perceptual changes	✖ Public education ✖ Environmental accommodations
Socio-Cultural	✖ Social skills ✖ Habit training ✖ Role playing ✖ Time management	✖ Role reorganization ✖ Value shifts ✖ Family therapy	✖ Role negotiation ✖ Social support ✖ Social network therapy
Environmental			✖ Human rights ✖ Adapted housing ✖ Transportation

transportation system more accessible so that Joe could participate in the mainstream of his community rather than being isolated in a disability "ghetto," where specialized services are the only option. This might involve joining with local senior citizens and disability groups to lobby for increased accessibility of local buses and commuter trains.

Although the intent of this book is not to delve into therapeutic applications of occupational therapy theory, the brief discussion in this chapter offers a few examples of how theory and practice interact. To this end, Table 14-1 looks at some of the therapeutic strategies and media that occupational therapists typically use. The table classifies these therapeutic approaches into the three types of strategies discussed in this chapter, while at the same time illustrating the area of theory upon which each depends.

Author Index

KEYWORD INDEX

This index directs the reader to bibliography entry numbers, not page numbers

General Index

Build Your Library

Along with this title, we publish numerous products on a variety of topics. We are sure that you will find the below titles to be an essential addition to your library. Order your copies today or contact us for a copy of our latest catalog for additional product information.

THEORETICAL BASIS OF OCCUPATIONAL THERAPY, SECOND EDITION

Mary Ann McColl PhD; Mary Law PhD, OT(C); Debra Stewart MSc, OT(C); Lorna Doubt MSc; Nancy Pollock MSc; and Terry Krupa PhD

208 pp., Soft Cover, 2002, ISBN 1-55642-540-6
Order #35406, **$34.95**

Significant developments in occupational therapy theory over the past 25 years are discussed in a user-friendly format. This exciting new edition begins with a discussion of the uses and applications of occupational therapy theory and offers ways of thinking about and organizing the theory. Perfect for the clinician or student, this necessary text contains volumes of information accessible in one convenient place.

MEASURING OCCUPATIONAL PERFORMANCE: SUPPORTING BEST PRACTICE IN OCCUPATIONAL THERAPY

Mary Law PhD, OT(C); Carolyn M. Baum PhD, OTR/C, FAOTA; and Winnie Dunn PhD, OTR, FAOTA

320 pp., Soft Cover, 2000, ISBN 1-55642-298-9
Order #32989, **$35.95**

This extraordinary text begins with a background of measurement concepts and issues and explores the central theoretical concept of occupational therapy, occupation, and occupational performance outcomes facilitated by person-environment-occupation. Measurement issues and practices are discussed, and a decision-making framework is provided to guide the choice of assessment tools.

EVIDENCE-BASED REHABILITATION: A GUIDE TO PRACTICE

Mary Law PhD, OT(C)

384 pp., Soft Cover, 2002, ISBN 1-55642-453-1, Order #44531, **$36.95**

Specifically written for rehabilitation practitioners, this exceptional text is not designed to teach students how to do research, but rather how to become critical consumers of research, therefore developing skills to ensure that their rehabilitation practice is based on the best evidence that is available. Much of the text focuses on how knowledge is developed, making it an essential tool for both students and practitioners.

Contact Us

SLACK Incorporated, Professional Book Division
6900 Grove Road, Thorofare, NJ 08086
1-800-257-8290/1-856-848-1000, Fax: 1-856-853-5991
orders@slackinc.com or www.slackbooks.com

ORDER FORM

QUANTITY	TITLE	ORDER #	PRICE
	Theoretical Basis of Occupational Therapy	35406	**$34.95**
	Measuring Occupational Performance	32989	**$35.95**
	Evidence-Based Rehabilitation: A Guide to Practice	44531	**$36.95**
		Subtotal	$
		Applicable state and local tax will be added to your purchase	$
		Handling	**$4.50**
		Total	$

Name: _____
Address: _____
City: _____ State: _____ Zip: _____
Phone: _____ Fax: _____
Email: _____

- Check enclosed (Payable to SLACK Incorporated)_____
- Charge my: ____ [card] ____ VISA ____ MasterCard

  Account #: _____
  Exp. date: _____ Signature: _____

NOTE: *Prices are subject to change without notice.*
Shipping charges will apply.
Shipping and handling charges are non-returnable.

CODE: 328